Practice-Based Learning & Improvement

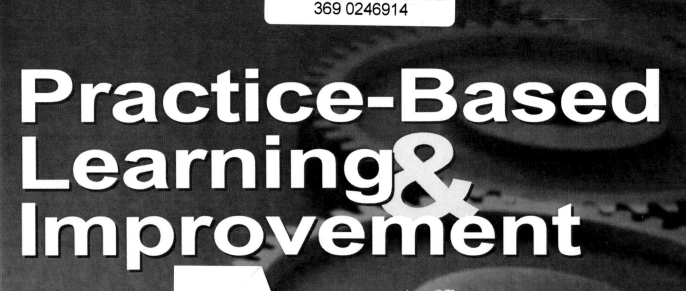

A Clinical Impr _____ *Action Guide*
Third Edition

This book is due

28 FEB

Edited by
Mark E. Splaine, M
Mary A. Dolansky, RN
Carlos A. Estrada, MD, MS
Patricia A. Patrician, PhD, RN, FAAN

Joint Commission Resources

Senior Editor: Lori Meek Schuldt
Contributing Editor: Steven Berman
Project Manager: Andrew Bernotas
Manager, Publications: Helen M. Fry, MA
Associate Director, Production: Johanna Harris
Executive Director: Catherine Chopp Hinckley, MA, PhD
Joint Commission Reviewers: Paul Schyve, MD, Senior Advisor, Healthcare Improvement, Division of Healthcare Improvement; Lon M. Berkeley, Co–Project Lead, Primary Care Medical Home Initiative, and Project Director, Community Health Center Accreditation; Belkys Teresa Gomez, RN, MSN, Associate Project Director–Specialist, Department of Standards and Survey Methods, Division of Healthcare Quality Evaluation; Joyce Webb, RN, MBA, CMPE, Project Director, Department of Standards and Survey Methods, Division of Healthcare Quality Evaluation

Joint Commission Resources Mission

The mission of Joint Commission Resources (JCR) is to continuously improve the safety and quality of health care in the United States and in the international community through the provision of education, publications, consultation, and evaluation services.

Joint Commission Resources educational programs and publications support, but are separate from, the accreditation activities of The Joint Commission. Attendees at Joint Commission Resources educational programs and purchasers of Joint Commission Resources publications receive no special consideration or treatment in, or confidential information about, the accreditation process.

The inclusion of an organization name, product, or service in a Joint Commission Resources publication should not be construed as an endorsement of such organization, product, or service, nor is failure to include an organization name, product, or service to be construed as disapproval.

Requests for permission to make copies of any part of this work should be mailed to
Permissions Editor
Department of Publications and Education
Joint Commission Resources
One Renaissance Boulevard
Oakbrook Terrace, Illinois 60181 U.S.A.
permissions@jcrinc.com

ISBN: 978-1-59940-707-4
Library of Congress Control Number: 2012950477

For more information about Joint Commission Resources, please visit http://www.jcrinc.com.

CONTENTS

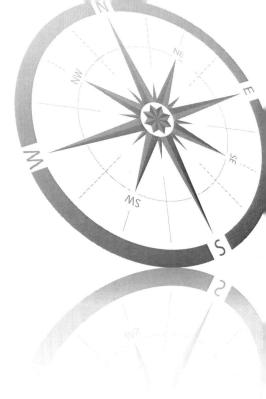

Contributors

Paul B. Batalden, MD, is Professor Emeritus of Pediatrics, Community and Family Medicine and The Dartmouth Institute for Health Policy and Clinical Practice at the Geisel School of Medicine at Dartmouth, Lebanon, New Hampshire.

Chaim M. Bell, MD, PhD, is Senior Quality Scholar at the University of Toronto site of the Veterans Affairs National Quality Scholars Fellowship Program and Associate Professor of Medicine and Health Policy, Management and Evaluation at the University of Toronto. He is Adjunct Scientist at the Institute for Clinical Evaluative Sciences and a Core Member of the University of Toronto Centre for Patient Safety, Toronto, Canada. He also holds a joint Canadian Institutes of Health Research and Canadian Patient Safety Institute Chair in Patient Safety and Continuity of Care.

Velinda Block, DNP, RN, NEA-BC, is Senior Associate Vice President and Chief Nursing Officer at the University of Alabama at Birmingham (UAB) University Hospital and Assistant Professor at the UAB School of Nursing.

Caitlin W. Brennan, RN, MSN, PhD, is Palliative Care Nurse Practitioner at the Veterans Affairs Boston Healthcare System, Boston, Massachusetts; and Postdoctoral Fellow at the Veterans Affairs National Quality Scholars Program at the Louis Stokes Cleveland Veterans Affairs Medical Center, Cleveland, Ohio.

Robert S. Dittus, MD, MPH, is the Albert and Bernard Werthan Professor of Medicine, Associate Vice Chancellor for Public Health and Health Care, Senior Associate Dean for Population Health Sciences, and Director, Institute for Medicine and Public Health, Vanderbilt University. He is Senior Quality Scholar of the Veterans Affairs National Quality Scholars Fellowship Program and Director, Geriatric Research, Education and Clinical Center at the Veterans Affairs Tennessee Valley Healthcare System, Nashville, Tennessee.

Mary A. Dolansky, PhD, RN, is Associate Professor at the Frances Payne Bolton School of Nursing, Case Western Reserve University, and Senior Quality Scholar of the Veterans Affairs National Quality Scholars Fellowship Program at the Louis Stokes Cleveland Veterans Affairs Medical Center, Cleveland, Ohio.

William H. Edwards, MD, is Professor and Vice Chair of Pediatrics, Neonatology Division Chief, and Section Chief, Neonatal Intensive Care Unit, Children's Hospital at Dartmouth-Hitchcock Medical Center, Lebanon, New Hampshire.

Carlos A. Estrada, MD, MS, is Senior Quality Scholar of the Veterans Affairs National Quality Scholars Fellowship Program at the Birmingham Veterans Affairs Medical Center and Professor of Medicine and Director of the Division of General Internal Medicine at the University of Alabama at Birmingham.

Deborah Gardner, PhD, RN, FNAP, FAAN, is former Senior Advisor at the Bureau of Health Professions, Health Resources and Services Administration, and Executive Director for the Hawaii State Center for Nursing in Honolulu.

Justin Glasgow, MS, is Affiliate Researcher at the Comprehensive Access and Delivery Research and Evaluation Center at the Iowa City Veterans Affairs Health Care System and an MD/PhD candidate at the University of Iowa Carver College of Medicine, Iowa City, Iowa.

Marjorie M. Godfrey, MS, RN, is Codirector of The Dartmouth Institute Microsystem Academy in the Center for Leadership and Improvement and Instructor in The Dartmouth Institute for Health Policy and Clinical Practice at the Geisel School of Medicine at Dartmouth, Lebanon, New Hampshire.

Julie K. Johnson, PhD, MSPH, is Deputy Director, Centre for Clinical Governance Research, and Associate Professor in the Faculty of Medicine at the University of New South Wales, Sydney, Australia.

Kimberly D. Johnson, RN, PhD, CEN, is Postdoctoral Fellow at the Veterans Affairs National Quality Scholars Fellowship Program at the Louis Stokes Cleveland Veterans Affairs Medical Center and Case Western Reserve University, Cleveland, Ohio.

Anne C. Jones, DO, is a family physician and Fellow at the Veterans Affairs National Quality Scholars Fellowship Program at the White River Junction Veterans Affairs Medical Center in White River Junction, Vermont. She is an Instructor in the Department of Community and Family Medicine at Geisel School of Medicine at Dartmouth and a Master of Public Health degree candidate at The Dartmouth Institute for Health Policy and Clinical Practice, Lebanon, New Hampshire.

Peter Kaboli, MD, MS, is Senior Quality Scholar at the Iowa City Veterans Affairs National Quality Scholars Fellowship Program and Investigator with the Center for Comprehensive Access and Delivery Research and Evaluation at the Iowa City Veterans Affairs Health Care System, and Professor of Internal Medicine, University of Iowa Carver College of Medicine, Iowa City, Iowa.

Maryjoan D. Ladden, PhD, RN, FAAN, is Senior Program Officer at the Robert Wood Johnson Foundation, Princeton, New Jersey.

Renée H. Lawrence, PhD, is Research Scientist at the Louis Stokes Cleveland Veterans Affairs Medical Center, Cleveland, Ohio.

Joel S. Lazar, MD, MPH, is Medical Director of Dartmouth Health Connect, Hanover, New Hampshire, and Assistant Professor, Community and Family Medicine and The Dartmouth Institute for Health Policy and Clinical Practice at the Geisel School of Medicine at Dartmouth, Lebanon, New Hampshire.

Connie Lopez, MSN, CNS, RNC-OB, CPHRM, is National Leader, Simulation-Based Education and Training, National Risk Management and Patient Safety, Kaiser Permanente Program Offices, Oakland, California.

Kieran P. McIntyre, MD, is Respirologist in the Department of Medicine at St. Michael's Hospital and is affiliated with the Toronto Adult Cystic Fibrosis Program. He is a graduate of the Veterans Affairs National Quality Scholars Fellowship Program at the University of Toronto, Toronto, Canada.

Rory F. McQuillan, MBBChBAO, MRCPI, is Nephrologist at the University Health Network and Fellow at the Veterans Affairs National Quality Scholars Fellowship Program at the University of Toronto, Toronto, Canada.

Rebecca S. Miltner, PhD, RN, is Assistant Professor at the University of Alabama at Birmingham School of Nursing. She is a graduate of the Veterans Affairs National Quality Scholars Fellowship Program.

Lorraine C. Mion, PhD, RN, FAAN, is the Independence Foundation Professor of Nursing at Vanderbilt University and Senior Quality Scholar of the Veterans Affairs National Quality Scholars Fellowship Program at the Veterans Affairs Tennessee Valley Health System, Nashville, Tennessee.

Anita D. Misra-Hebert, MD, FACP, is Assistant Professor of Medicine at Cleveland Clinic Lerner College of Medicine, Case Western Reserve University, and Fellow at the Veterans Affairs National Quality Scholars Fellowship Program at the Louis Stokes Cleveland Veterans Affairs Medical Center, Cleveland, Ohio.

Shirley M. Moore, PhD, RN, FAAN, is Associate Dean for Research and the Edward J. and Louise Mellen Professor of Nursing at the Frances Payne Bolton School of Nursing at Case Western Reserve University, Cleveland, Ohio, and Nursing Leader of the Veterans Affairs National Quality Scholars Fellowship Program.

Eugene C. Nelson, DSc, MPH, is Associate Director of the Center for Population Health at The Dartmouth Institute (TDI) for Health Policy and Clinical Practice. He is Professor in TDI and Community and Family Medicine at the Geisel School of Medicine at Dartmouth, Lebanon, New Hampshire.

Jeremiah H. Newsom, MD, MSPH, is Hospitalist at Ochsner Medical Center, New Orleans, Louisiana. He is a graduate of the Veterans Affairs National Quality Scholars Fellowship Program.

Greg Ogrinc, MD, MS, is Senior Scholar at the Veterans Affairs National Quality Scholars Fellowship Program in White River Junction, Vermont, Director of the Health Systems and Clinical Improvement Program, and Associate Professor of Community and Family Medicine and of Medicine at the Geisel School of Medicine at Dartmouth in Hanover, New Hampshire.

Danielle M. Olds, RN, MPH, PhD, is a Fellow at the Veterans Affairs National Quality Scholars Fellowship Program at the Louis Stokes Cleveland Veterans Affairs Medical Center and Postdoctoral Fellow at the Frances Payne Bolton School of Nursing, Case Western Reserve University, Cleveland, Ohio.

Patricia A. Patrician, PhD, RN, FAAN, is Associate Professor and Donna Brown Banton Endowed Professor at the University of Alabama at Birmingham School of Nursing and Senior Quality Scholar of the Veterans Affairs National Quality Scholars Fellowship Program, Birmingham Veterans Affairs Medical Center, Birmingham, Alabama.

Robert M. Patrick, MD, MBA, is Hospitalist and Fellow, Veterans Affairs National Quality Scholars Fellowship Program at the Louis Stokes Cleveland Veterans Affairs Medical Center, Cleveland, Ohio.

Grant T. Savage, PhD, is Codirector of the Healthcare Leadership Academy and Professor of Management in the School of Business, University of Alabama at Birmingham.

Tracy Shamburger, PhD, RN, is former Healthcare Associated Infection Coordinator, Alabama Department of Public Health, and Major, Officer in Charge of Education and Training, 908th United States Air Force Reserves, Montgomery, Alabama. She is a Fellow at the Veterans Affairs National Quality Scholars Fellowship Program at the Birmingham Veterans Affairs Medical Center and the University of Alabama at Birmingham.

Mamta K. Singh, MD, MS, is Codirector for the Center for Excellence in Primary Care Education at the Louis Stokes Cleveland Veterans Affairs Medical Center, Director of Patient Based Programs, and Associate Professor of Medicine at Case Western Reserve University School of Medicine, Cleveland, Ohio.

Mark E. Splaine, MD, MS, is Director of Educational Programs at The Dartmouth Institute (TDI) for Health Policy and Clinical Practice and Director of the Veterans Affairs National Quality Scholars Fellowship Program. He is an Associate Professor in TDI and Community and Family Medicine at the Geisel School of Medicine at Dartmouth, Lebanon, New Hampshire.

Benjamin B. Taylor, MD, MPH, is Chief Quality Officer, University of Alabama at Birmingham (UAB) University Hospital, Assistant Professor of Medicine at UAB, and Associate Fellowship Director at the Birmingham Veterans Affairs National Quality Scholars Fellowship Program, Birmingham, Alabama.

Jennifer D. Thull-Freedman, MD, MSc, is Director of Quality and Patient Safety in the Division of Pediatric Emergency Medicine at Alberta Children's Hospital and Clinical Associate Professor at the University of Calgary. She is a graduate of the Veterans Affairs National Quality Scholars Fellowship Program at the University of Toronto, Toronto, Canada.

Michael A. Tijerina, RN-BC, BSN, is Professional Development Consultant, National Patient Care Services, Kaiser Permanente, Oakland, California, and Adjunct Faculty for the California Simulation Alliance instructor training program.

Alene A. Toulany, MD, FRCPC, is a Fellow in the Division of Adolescent Medicine at the Hospital for Sick Children and University of Toronto, and a Fellow at the Veterans Affairs National Quality Scholars Fellowship Program at the University of Toronto, Toronto, Canada.

Brook Watts, MD, MS, is Chief Quality Officer at the Louis Stokes Cleveland Veterans Affairs Medical Center and Associate Professor of Medicine at Case Western Reserve University, Cleveland, Ohio.

Robert Weech-Maldonado, PhD, MBA, is Professor and L.R. Jordan Endowed Chair, Department of Health Services Administration at the University of Alabama at Birmingham.

David E. Willens, MD, MPH, is Associate Program Director for Internal Medicine Residency and a Quality Improvement Specialist for the Division of General Internal Medicine at Henry Ford Health System, Detroit, Michigan. He is a graduate of the Veterans Affairs National Quality Scholars Fellowship Program.

Acknowledgment and Disclaimer

The Department of Veterans Affairs National Quality Scholars Fellowship Program (VAQS) is funded by the Department of Veterans Affairs Office of Academic Affiliations (OAA). The opinions expressed in this book are those of the contributing authors alone and do not necessarily reflect the views, opinions, or policies of the Department of Veterans Affairs.

Foreword

WORKPLACE LEARNING

Shirley M. Moore

Workplace learning. One of the hallmarks of a professional is the commitment to continual self-growth and learning. This book has as its premise that the workplace of health professionals is a vast laboratory for learning and improving—improving ourselves as professionals, improving the care we personally provide, and improving the quality and efficiency of the health care delivery system. *Practice-Based Learning and Improvement: A Clinical Improvement Action Guide* is about workplace learning. It addresses the frontline clinician's role in simultaneously providing care and improving it.

Fortunately, there is a process of how to go about workplace learning. It is the use of continuous quality improvement methodology. Quality improvement methods constitute a *learning infrastructure* for the practice workplace. Just as we have infrastructure supports for other aspects of our workplace (managing human resources, billing, administrative procedures, and so on), we can set up infrastructure support to ensure learning and improvement. Learning infrastructures do not leave learning to chance[1]; they provide systematic opportunities to reflect on and improve care. Engaging in workplace learning requires the clinician to adopt a "learning stance" toward the care provided in the practice organization, which means temporarily suspending the view of oneself as "expert" and taking on the attitude of a "learner"—that is, someone who openly seeks greater understanding of and improvement in the workplace.

Peter Senge, author of *The Fifth Discipline*, states that individuals must collaborate with others in the workplace to form learning teams and work in learning cycles.[1] These professional learning teams identify problems or issues, gather relevant data, test solutions in the workplace "laboratory," evaluate the results, and harvest the most suitable solutions for application. This process is effective for finding new solutions to old problems and for enabling care systems to be flexible and responsive to changing needs. These workplace teams learn through the process of continual movement between practice and reflection on practice, which promotes higher performance in the short term while building a learning culture for the long term.

Workplace learning also creates the opportunity to experience more joy in our daily work. In addition to the joy of improving outcomes associated with our work—enhanced health status of our patients and greater quality and efficiency in our delivery systems—the use of quality improvement methods allows us to experience the positive attributes associated with learning, such as creativity, aspiration, inquiry, and dialogue.

A major goal of this book is to reduce the abstract idea of practice-based learning and improvement down to a set of concrete activities. Practice-based learning and improvement is a skill-based activity with theoretical underpinnings.[2] These skills and examples of their application are described in this action guide. So, when someone asks you, "Just what is practice-based learning and improvement, anyway?" a straightforward response is that it is workplace learning. It is about continually seeking to understand

and change your workplace to improve care. Practice-based learning and improvement is not conceptually difficult to understand. It is a culture, a process, and a set of tools that when embedded into your practice support workplace learning.

References

1. Senge PM. *The Fifth Discipline: The Art and Practice of the Learning Organization.* New York: Doubleday, 2006.
2. Ogrinc G, et al. Teaching and assessing resident competence in practice-based learning and improvement. *J Gen Intern Med.* 2004 May;19(5 Pt 2):496–500.

Introduction

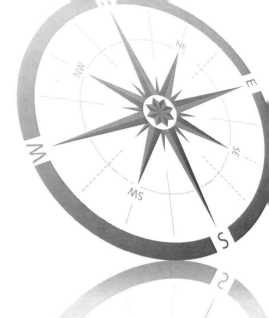

The Context in Which We Live and Practice

**Mark E. Splaine, Eugene C. Nelson, Paul B. Batalden,
Mary A. Dolansky, Carlos A. Estrada, Patricia A. Patrician**

Every health professional knows—as does every patient, every loved one, every participant in the process of care—that health care can be improved.

Although we know this, as health professionals, we likely received little if any formal training in improvement methods during our education, nor was the expectation of continuous quality improvement work built explicitly into our job descriptions. We know it as recipients of those same health services, although as patients we probably trust and respect our own providers, who are committed to the relief of our suffering and the promotion of our well-being.

We know it, ultimately, because we have experienced in our professional or personal lives the significant gap between what is possible in modern medicine and what in reality often transpires. Indeed, despite the talents and compassion and best intentions of all participants, we deliver, receive, or manage clinical service in systems that have not been designed for best care. Abundant data now support this assertion. The original work in this area began coming to light in 2000 when the Institute of Medicine (IOM) issued its report *To Err Is Human: Building a Safer Health System.*[1] The report documented nearly 100,000 needless health care system–related deaths in the United States per year. Since then, several studies over time have demonstrated repeatedly that Americans receive only 40% to 60% of recommended interventions for acute, chronic, and preventive care needs.[2-4] The IOM concluded in its 2001 report *Crossing the Quality Chasm* that significant deficiencies in the design of our current system consistently undermine delivery of the highest-quality care.[5] Despite the fact that these issues have been known for more than 10 years, only some progress has been made in making the whole health care system better and safer.

These IOM reports demand our attention at a time when other important health care developments create "tension for change"[6] as well. In recent years, for example, institutional and even individual practitioner measures of health care quality, safety, and cost have been made increasingly transparent to patients, payers, and the public. In 2003 and 2004 the National Quality Forum called for public release of quality and safety measures by hospitals, nursing homes, and other health care providers.[7] Moreover, the Centers for Medicare & Medicaid Services (CMS) and The Joint Commission have mandated public reporting by hospitals of core quality measures pertinent to common health conditions and patient perceptions.[8]

In parallel with this transition to increased transparency, health care payment systems continue to move in the direction of "value-based purchasing" to reward higher quality and lower costs. Private insurers and now Medicare continue to base reimbursement for chronic disease management on providers' measurable compliance with evidence-based quality recommendations, and trends toward value-based purchasing of health services will certainly continue.[9] The model of Accountable Care Organizations (ACOs) that has been adopted by CMS was a further manifestation of this development.[10] In addition, the signing of the Patient Protection and Affordable Care Act into law in 2010 is a further step in the direction of national health care reform.[11] Moreover, metrics for both quality and cost will grow more accurate and pervasive, so that informed patients might selectively entrust their care and informed purchasers can selectively channel their beneficiaries to health care organizations that deliver highest value.

During this time, the Accreditation Council for Graduate Medical Education (ACGME) clarified and expanded the expected skill sets of physicians and mandated the explicit building of these skills into professional education. In 1999 ACGME officially endorsed six general competencies that all graduates of board-certified residency programs must master: patient care, medical knowledge, professionalism, systems-based practice, interpersonal and communication skills, and (notably) practice-based learning and improvement.[12] Undergraduate and graduate medical training programs have developed formal tracking systems to document achievement of these competency goals, and continuing education for practicing physicians will increasingly target these goals as well. Likewise, the American Board of Medical Specialties (ABMS) adopted similar competencies for all practicing physicians, which are to be demonstrated through maintenance of certification.[13]

In addition, the national project Quality and Safety Education for Nurses, sponsored by the Robert Wood Johnson Foundation, has developed comparable competencies for nurses across the spectrum of nursing education and practice (prelicensure and graduate).[14] These competencies include patient-centered care, teamwork and collaboration, evidence-based practice, quality improvement, safety, and informatics. The Quality Improvement competency articulates that nurses develop the knowledge, skills, and attitudes to "use data to monitor the outcomes of care processes and use improvement methods to design and test changes to continuously improve the quality and safety of health care systems."[14] This competency is similar to the Practice-Based Learning and Improvement competency described by the ACGME and ABMS.

The imperative to achieve better clinical outcomes, to improve system performance, and to build improvement knowledge into professional training and development is more critical than ever.[15] The time is here to explicitly work to better connect system improvement with both clinical practice and clinical learning. Through such efforts, we can add value to the care we offer our patients, and we can increase satisfaction in our own professional lives.

The Purpose of This Book

For this third edition of this text, we are once again motivated by the vision to develop a culture of quality in health care systems, and we endeavor in *Practice-Based Learning and Improvement: A Clinical Improvement Action Guide* to empower health professionals to realize this vision in their own practices. We assume from the outset (and reiterate throughout this edition) that quality improvement is the work of everyone and that it must be directed simultaneously to the mutually supportive goals of better clinical outcomes, better system performance, and better professional training and development.

To support these goals, we offer both a conceptual framework and practical tools, and we combine the two in exercises and case studies that challenge the reader to identify local resources and opportunities, to define improvement tasks more precisely, and to act, so that positive and meaningful change becomes synonymous with clinical work itself.

Because quality improvement is indeed the work of everyone, the editors and the authors of each chapter draw from experts in both nursing and medicine to ensure that multiple health professional perspectives are represented. Further, we have developed this book with several audiences in mind—clinicians, teachers and mentors of clinicians, participants of interdisciplinary work groups, and leaders of health care programs and systems. Clinicians will discover practical improvement tools that are designed for use in a variety of settings. The Clinical Value Compass in particular will support practitioners' identification of worthy goals for improvement, clarification of target measures, analysis and benchmarking of current practice patterns, and design of specific tests of local change. Educators can adapt these same ideas and instruments for didactic purposes and can apply specific principles and methods to develop action-based training modules for learners at any level of health professional development. Interdisciplinary work groups will find similar support for their educational and improvement projects, with special attention to strategies and techniques that build upon the unique knowledge and skills of all participants. Health care leaders will recognize the applicability of value compass thinking in management settings, where it can stimulate structured planning and implementation of new initiatives and facilitate monitoring of balanced outcome measures in domains of patient care quality, health care costs, and system performance.

The Design and Use of This Book

We invite readers to join us on a journey of both action and reflection. Although busy health professionals might choose to "sample" individual chapters that are relevant to specific concerns, *Practice-Based Learning and Improvement: A Clinical Improvement Action Guide* is constructed with a developmental trajectory in mind. Beginning in Chapter 1 and proceeding in order through Chapter 6, we move from the general to the specific, and then, in Chapters 7 through 9, "circle back," after simpler concepts have been mastered, to higher-order syntheses with more general application. In this manner, we hope to track the natural progression of action-based learning, and we encourage readers to follow the same path. Health professionals who are new to the field might thus wish to dedicate more time to the basic principles of early chapters (1 through 6), while practitioners with greater quality improvement experience might proceed more quickly to the advanced discussion in the later chapters (7 through 9).

Chapter 1 introduces essential knowledge systems that support the work of practice-based learning and improvement. This conceptual framework establishes relevant context for the more task-oriented chapters that follow. Improvement work itself begins in Chapter 2, and with it the process of practice-based learning in local contexts of care. We lead the reader through a brainstorming exercise that generates multiple new ideas for

improvement, building up resources available to all of us in our daily work. In Chapter 3, these ideas are refined and made operational. The Clinical Improvement Worksheet is introduced to guide both individual practitioners and work groups in identifying and targeting specific aims and in developing specific tests of change that support measurable and sustainable improvement in both processes and outcomes of care.

The Clinical Value Compass, described in detail in Chapter 4, is a conceptual and practical centerpiece of practice-based learning and improvement, and indeed its "arrows" point both backward and forward to the other chapters. We focus here on measuring what matters most: patient outcomes. But we define these outcomes in balanced terms that honor not only clinical or biologic parameters but also measures of functional status, patient perception and satisfaction, and cost. Case studies demonstrate the utility of the Clinical Value Compass in clarifying and measuring outcomes in all these important domains.

In Chapter 5, we turn attention outward from local contexts of care and introduce benchmarking techniques that facilitate scanning of the external environment for comparative practice patterns. The chapter's benchmarking worksheet can be used in concert with the Clinical Value Compass to answer the following important questions:

- Who is getting the best outcomes?
- What are they doing to get those best outcomes?
- What does the evidence base tell us about achieving outcomes of similar quality?

We also describe the method of Achievable Benchmarks of Care as an example of a published approach to benchmarking that has demonstrated results in improving care.[16]

Chapter 6 invites readers to explore change concepts that direct attention to high-leverage improvement opportunities. We consider 10 core concepts that have proven particularly valuable in our own work, and we demonstrate their applicability in an extended case study.

Subsequent chapters broaden and deepen the scope of both action and understanding in practice-based learning and improvement. Chapter 7 focuses on implementing, spreading, and sustaining organizational change. It builds specifically on Chapters 2 and 6 and provides readers with an in-depth exploration of the Institute for Healthcare Improvement's Framework for Spread as well as examples of successful organizational change efforts in health care settings.

In Chapter 8 we focus on health professional involvement in practice-based learning and improvement. It builds on all the preceding chapters by emphasizing that every aspect of practice-based learning and improvement is done in teams of health professionals and usually with learners of some type. Specifically, this chapter provides readers with an overview of the importance of teamwork and collaboration for both organizational leaders and health care workers; a review of effective components of teamwork and strategies to increase collaboration as well as interprofessional education and its core competencies; and examples from a large integrated health care delivery system on programs for team training and training techniques and resources.

Chapter 9 represents the culmination of the concepts built up through the first eight chapters. It demonstrates how the patient-centered medical home model can fully incorporate the concept of practice-based learning and improvement. Readers are invited to consider two examples from different organizations to visualize the alignment and consider how to make use of this approach in their own context.

We include a series of appendixes to support the adaptation of concepts and methods to the local settings:

- Appendix A provides a full set of improvement worksheets for use by individual practitioners or improvement teams.
- Appendix B describes observational methods to include in quality improvement and provides interview worksheets specifically adapted for application in improvement efforts.
- Appendix C describes a compilation of patient-reported measures of quality and value and provides links to a number of resources to access additional information about these measures.

- Appendix D outlines 9 principles for using data in clinical practice for learning and improvement and includes guidelines with 12 suggestions for designing a measurement process.
- Appendix E provides a starter set of websites that can further stimulate and support practice-based learning and improvement efforts.
- Appendix F provides additional material from Chapter 8 to enhance readers' understanding of resources for health professional involvement in practice-based learning and improvement.
- Appendix G lists examples of Web-based resources for education related to quality and patient safety that can support efforts to learn about and apply ideas for practice-based learning and improvement.
- Appendix H summarizes the Standards for Quality Improvement Reporting Excellence (SQUIRE) Guidelines. These guidelines can be used in planning practice-based learning and improvement, regardless of whether the goal is to report the work in the literature.

Summary

We invite readers to draw on the ideas put forward in this text, to reflect on familiar patterns of practice, to acknowledge local barriers to quality care, and to recognize local resources (human and material) that can support and sustain improvement. Those resources are in fact abundant. Our hope is that this book will be counted among them and, more important, that it will stimulate readers to engage all resources in a new and more effective manner. The result, we believe, will be a new appreciation of the job of everyone, the simultaneous doing and improving of our work. Not only our patients but also we ourselves will benefit from this worthy effort.

References

1. Kohn LT, Corrigan JM, Donaldson MS; Committee on Quality of Health Care in America, Institute of Medicine. *To Err Is Human: Building a Safer Health System.* Washington, DC: National Academy Press, 2000.
2. McGlynn EA, et al. The quality of health care delivered to adults in the United States. *N Engl J Med.* 2003 Jun 26;348(26):2635–2645.

3. Asch SM, et al. Who is at greatest risk for receiving poor-quality health care? *N Engl J Med.* 2006 Mar 16(11);354:1147–1156.

4. Mangione-Smith R, et al. The quality of ambulatory care delivered to children in the United States. *N Engl J Med.* 2007 Oct 11;357(15):1515–1523.

5. Committee on Quality of Health Care in America, Institute of Medicine. *Crossing the Quality Chasm: A New Health System for the 21st Century.* Washington, DC: National Academy Press, 2001.

6. Gustafson DH, Cats-Baril WL, Alemi F. *Systems to Support Health Policy Analysis: Theory, Models, and Uses.* Ann Arbor, MI: Health Administration Press, 1992.

7. National Quality Forum. Reports. [Link no longer active] http://www.qualityforum.org/publications/reports.

8. The Joint Commission. Performance Measurement Initiatives. [Link no longer active] http://www.jointcommission.org/PerformanceMeasurement/PerformanceMeasurement.

9. Trude S, Au M, Christianson JB. Health plan pay-for-performance strategies. *Am J Manag Care.* 2006 Sep;12(9):537–542.

10. Center for Medicare & Medicaid Services. Accountable Care Organizations (ACO). (Updated: Apr 5, 2012.) Accessed Oct 13, 2012. https://www.cms.gov/Medicare/Medicare-Fee-for-Service-Payment/ACO/index.html?redirect=/ACO.

11. HealthCare.gov. The Health Care Law & You. Accessed Oct 13, 2012. http://www.healthcare.gov/law/index.html.

12. Accreditation Council for Graduate Medical Education. ACGME Outcome Project: Competencies. [Link no longer active] http://www.acgme.org/outcome/comp/compHome.asp.

13. American Board of Medical Specialties. MOC Competencies and Criteria. Accessed Oct 13, 2012. http://www.abms.org/maintenance_of_certification/MOC_competencies.aspx.

14. Quality and Safety Education for Nurses. Quality and Safety Competencies. Accessed Oct 13, 2012. http://www.qsen.org/competencies.php.

15. Batalden PB, Davidoff F. What is "quality improvement" and how can it transform health care? *Qual Saf Health Care.* 2007 Feb;16(1):2–3.

16. Weissman NW, et al. Achievable benchmarks of care: The ABC™s of benchmarking. *J Eval Clin Pract.* 1999 Aug;5(3):269–281.

Chapter 1

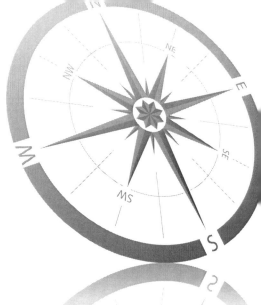

UNDERSTANDING CLINICAL IMPROVEMENT: FOUNDATIONS OF KNOWLEDGE FOR CHANGE IN HEALTH CARE SYSTEMS

Danielle M. Olds, Caitlin W. Brennan, Anita D. Misra-Hebert, Kimberly D. Johnson, Robert M. Patrick, Joel S. Lazar, Eugene C. Nelson, Paul B. Batalden

Quality is not an act. It is a habit.
          —Aristotle (384 BC–322 BC)[1(p. 31)]

The health care landscape has changed dramatically since the early 1990s. The findings of the Harvard Medical Practice Study in 1991[2,3] raised considerable awareness of the extent of errors and adverse events, but it was the release of the Institute of Medicine report *To Err Is Human* in 2000[4] that catalyzed a much broader interest in health care quality and safety. Since that time, in the United States, health care facilities, regions, states, and the federal government have worked toward health care improvement. These efforts have ranged from public reporting of quality measures to payment reform to education and partnership initiatives. States, such as New York and Pennsylvania, are reporting hospital performance on a variety of metrics in an effort to increase transparency and competition.[5] The US Centers for Medicare & Medicaid Services (CMS) also publicly reports hospital quality measures through the Hospital Compare website.[6] CMS payment reforms have included nonreimbursement of hospitals for the additional costs incurred for certain errors (so-called never events)[7] and the Hospital Value-Based Purchasing program, in which hospitals can receive incentive payments for meeting certain performance measures.[8] The Patient Protection and Affordable Care Act of 2010 established the CMS Innovation Center. The goal of the center is to find new ways of paying for and delivering high-quality care while decreasing costs. One strategy to meet this goal is the Health Care Innovation Awards. The first awards were granted in May 2012 to 26 organizations implementing innovative delivery models designed to lower health care spending.[9] National health care improvement efforts are not limited to the United States. The United Kingdom has the National Health Service Institute for Innovation and Improvement. The goal of the institute is to improve health care through innovation in areas such as the patient experience; population health; productivity and efficiency; safety; and adoption of health care change.[10]

Yet despite all these initiatives, quality improvement still begins with health professionals connecting their scientific knowledge to daily work patterns and embracing opportunities for practice-based learning. This chapter introduces a framework for understanding clinical quality and practice-based learning and continuous improvement as represented in real-world health care settings. We begin by presenting an example of two patients* who received contrasting levels of care for their chronic conditions. We explore the foundations of quality improvement in clinical practice,

---

* Although examples in this book are based on actual experiences, names of all patients are fictitious.

with attention to an understanding of the systems that are required for optimization of patient care, and we emphasize the evolving nature of health outcomes that are the final measure of this care. Discussions of continuous quality improvement must be grounded in the reality of clinicians' daily work and directed to the priorities of individual patients; in this chapter we introduce the supporting language and concepts for these discussions.

Two Patients with High Blood Glucose Levels: The Need to Close the Gaps

Patient 1

Mr. Clarke, a man in his late 40s, presented to the emergency department with a blood glucose level over 500 mg/dL. He had been diagnosed with diabetes six years prior, when he was initially treated with insulin and then was switched to oral medications after his blood glucose levels became better controlled. However, he admitted to recently not having followed his diet and exercise regimens as closely as before, and he had gained about 30 pounds during the past year. He felt thirsty and tired and remembered this feeling being classified as a symptom when his diabetes was first diagnosed. He was treated acutely, and the nurse set up a follow-up appointment with his primary care physician.

Mr. Clarke's follow-up appointment was at a newly established patient-centered medical home (PCMH). The PCMH is a team-based health care delivery model led by a physician that provides comprehensive and continuous care to patients. The health care team had access to his emergency visit records through a shared electronic health record system. The physician talked with Mr. Clarke about the difficulties he had in following his diet and exercise routines and provided approaches for better self-management. She prescribed insulin and referred him to a diabetes nurse educator and a pharmacist for further education. Before Mr. Clarke left the appointment, he was able to see the diabetes nurse educator, who reinforced the diet and exercise plan and verified that he knew how to administer his insulin. The nurse in the office documented

the patient's plan through the electronic health record system to ensure that the team was aware of the plan and would be prepared for his next appointment. A week later when Mr. Clarke met with the pharmacist, he was feeling better and his blood glucose levels were well controlled. At a one-month follow-up PCMH appointment, the physician reviewed recent lab values with Mr. Clark and noted that they were much improved. In addition, she reviewed the medication regimen, and Mr. Clark was again counseled by the diabetes nurse educator about his diet and exercise goals to strategize ways to overcome future barriers.

Patient 2

Mr. Jarvis, a man in his late 30s, presented to an internist's office with a chief complaint of feeling thirsty. He had a history of asthma and was overweight. He had recently been to an emergency department because of an asthma exacerbation and had been placed on treatment, including oral prednisone. The emergency department was not affiliated with the internist's office and had no access to any records of his specific treatment to review. As the physician obtained a detailed history from the patient, Mr. Jarvis recalled that he had been told he had "borderline" diabetes one year before, when he was hospitalized for asthma, but was told no other treatment was needed at that time. He had not checked his blood glucose recently. His blood glucose level was 380 mg/dL during the office visit, which confirmed a new diagnosis of diabetes. The physician ordered additional blood and urine tests and prescribed a medication. Mr. Jarvis reported that he did not have a primary care provider. Mr. Jarvis was scheduled for an appointment with the diabetes nurse educator and was asked to return the following week.

When considering Mr. Clarke and Mr. Jarvis, which factors will affect how "healthy" they will be in the next 10 years?

Mr. Clarke is supported with access to a well-functioning, interprofessional clinical care system and a team-based approach to controlling his diabetes. His providers work as an interprofessional team. If he is satisfied with the care he receives and maintains a regular source of care, he may be more likely to remain healthy. The major barrier to Mr. Clarke's diabetes control—and a measurable improvement in clinical parameters such as glycosolated hemoglobin (A1C) or prevention of diabetes complications—may be his own motivation to modify his health-related choices, coupled with the broader environmental and social context of where he lives, his socioeconomic status, and the strength of his social support systems. A quality challenge is to determine how successful his providers are at supporting his self-efficacy within this environmental and social context and to evaluate how to measure the complex interchange of these factors.

In contrast, Mr. Jarvis has not had a regular source of care. He now has two chronic diseases that have required urgent care. The fact that he had to seek emergency treatment for his asthma may be an indicator of suboptimal disease management; in addition, he was seen at an emergency department unaffiliated with the clinic where he later presented for care. The providers who treated him in the emergency department for asthma likely also possessed the necessary scientific knowledge about diabetes and knew that prescribing a steroid such as prednisone could raise blood glucose levels. The patient, however, may not have mentioned that he had previously been told that he had "borderline" diabetes, and there were no prior medical records available for review that documented this history. Thus, prescribing the steroid may have occurred without full information regarding the context of Mr. Jarvis's case. Mr. Jarvis then sought care for his symptom of thirst at a different facility, received care from a provider with whom he was not familiar, received a new diagnosis of a chronic disease, and was asked to follow up at a later date. He too may have barriers related to self-efficacy, but uncoordinated care—a pattern that is likely to continue for this patient—may contribute more immediately to worsened outcomes and increased risk for complications related to both his diabetes and his asthma. The quality challenge is for Mr. Jarvis's health care providers to change the system of care so that it delivers an organized, interprofessional approach to disease management.

Foundations of Continuous Quality Improvement and Practice-Based Learning

If our goal is to improve the care of patients in real-world clinical settings and to achieve this improvement in the context of real-world constraints on available resources, then we must commit ourselves to a process of reflection and learning that occurs in the "real time" of clinical practice itself. This process begins with an exploration of essential components in the work of quality improvement. Four foundational concepts require special attention: the functionality of systems and microsystems of care, the use of the Clinical Improvement Formula, the priority of clinical outcomes, and the necessity of viewing quality improvement as the work of everyone. The remainder of this chapter explores these four concepts in detail.

Systems and Microsystems of Care

Neither patient care nor quality improvement should be played as a "solo sport" in the twenty-first century. In both clinical endeavors and quality improvement, the challenge and the opportunity to health care professionals are to sustain both individual and collective competence, a cumulative whole of knowledge, skills, and experience. The efficacy of both clinical organizations and quality improvement teams derives in large part from the capacity of individuals to work together in—and as—well-integrated systems of care.

When Mr. Clarke and Mr. Jarvis experienced care for their chronic conditions, they joined company in their respective health care journeys not with isolated clinicians but with sequential professional members of clinical teams, as well as with members of multiple teams. The points of transition between members of each team and between the teams themselves were critical moments in the determination of overall quality of care. The emergency department evaluation; the communication between clinicians and administrative staff; the discharge instructions; and the coordination of outpatient follow-up, including the primary care provider, pharmacist, and diabetes nurse educator—each of these transitional steps shifted performance responsibility to a new clinical team in Mr. Clarke's and Mr. Jarvis's ongoing care.

There is great utility in identifying these smaller working groups as the true functional units of clinical care. Such groups (of people, information, and technology) are referred to as *clinical microsystems*[11]—the small, naturally occurring frontline units that provide most clinical care to most people. Clinical microsystems are highly interprofessional. These units can be characterized in terms of functional processes, patterns of communication, and the skill sets of each participant. They can also be understood organizationally, in relation to both the patients they serve and the larger health care systems of which they are a part.

As depicted in Figure 1-1 on page 5, microsystems can be conceptualized as one of several levels in an expanding series of health services and determinants. At the center of any health system is the individual or family with an active health need. Successive rings in the figure depict the patient in relationship with a clinician—whether a physician, nurse, or other trained provider—and then with the clinical microsystem itself, where patients, clinicians, and health care teams meet. Microsystems are supported in turn by larger mesosystems and macrosystems of care, which themselves are embedded in an economic, regulatory, and cultural environment that influences all levels of the health care system. These relationships are further characterized as follows:

- **Microsystems Are the Foundations of Patients' Experiences in the Health Care System.** In their respective journeys, Mr. Clarke and Mr. Jarvis moved through numerous microsystems of care. The emergency department, primary care office, and other providers (including a diabetes nurse educator, a pharmacist, and a dietitian) were not only physical settings, the background against which health and illness were experienced, but also active players. These settings and players are thought of as the "sharp end" of the health care system where quality, safety, satisfaction, and costs are continually created.[12(p.10)] These domains are described

in greater detail in subsequent sections and chapters as part of a model called the Clinical Value Compass. Clinical outcomes depend on what patients, such as Mr. Clarke and Mr. Jarvis, bring to each microsystem (for example, relevant information, prior health status, genetic endowment) and on what each microsystem does to (or with) that same patient (assessment, diagnosis, treatment, monitoring, and follow-up), as shown in Figure 1-2 (page 5).

- **Microsystems Are Linked, Tightly or Loosely, with Other Clinical Microsystems.** Collections of microsystems (for example, a paramedic team, an emergency department, an inpatient unit, and a primary care practice) form mesosystems of care that serve patients with specific needs (for example, cardiac, obstetric, oncologic, or pediatric care). Relationships within this greater mesosystem, as within the microsystem units themselves, might be implicit or explicit, where specific functional processes, patterns of communication, and participant competencies determine the overall quality of care that is provided.

- **Microsystems Are Often Embedded in Larger Macrosystems.** Frontline clinical units are often components of larger health systems (that is, macrosystems) that share common oversight and administrative infrastructure, such as hospitals, group practices, or networks of health care facilities. The microsystem relies on this larger macrosystem to provide clinical and administrative supports that are essential to both patient care and business operations. Such supports might include diagnostic testing, health records management, transportation, pharmacy, billing, and informatics coordination. The large health system, in turn, depends on clinical microsystems to deliver the "product"—in this case, to provide the right care in the right way at the right time.

The Clinical Improvement Formula

Experienced clinicians are well practiced in the art and skill of contextualizing scientific evidence—

Figure 1-1. The Relationship of Smaller and Larger Systems in Health Care: Systems Embedded in Systems

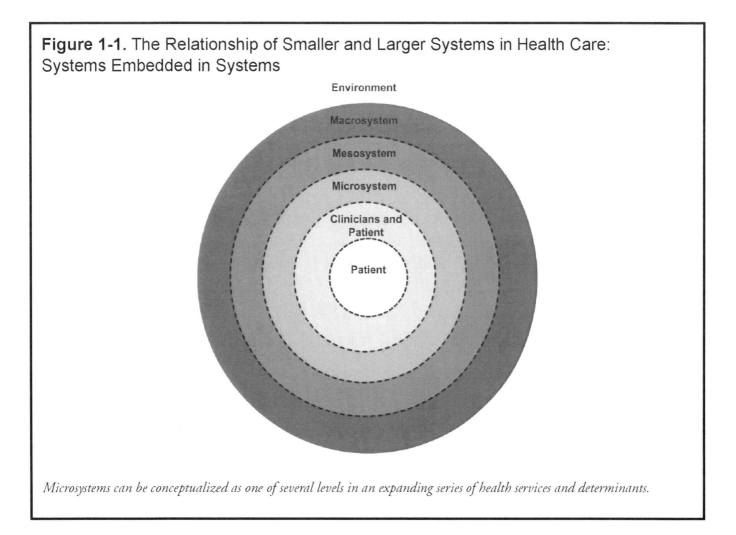

Microsystems can be conceptualized as one of several levels in an expanding series of health services and determinants.

Figure 1-2. Clinical Microsystem Linkages for Two Chronic Disease Patients on Their Health Care Journeys

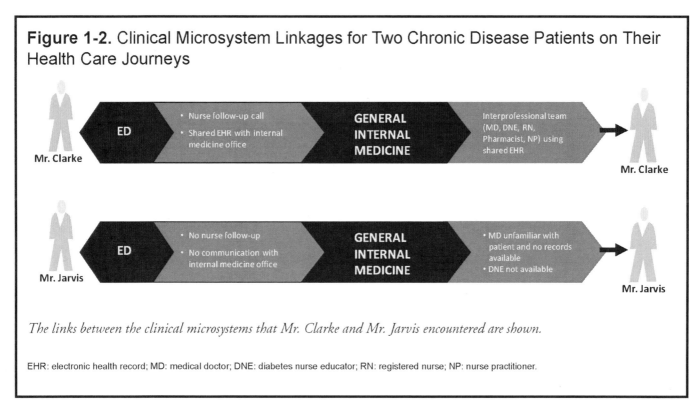

The links between the clinical microsystems that Mr. Clarke and Mr. Jarvis encountered are shown.

EHR: electronic health record; MD: medical doctor; DNE: diabetes nurse educator; RN: registered nurse; NP: nurse practitioner.

adapting general (and generic) recommendations to the unique needs, preferences, and capabilities of individual patients and then monitoring the specific effects of this adaptation: "How does that clinical guideline apply to this patient in the office with me today?" Similar forms of translation and adaptation support continuous quality improvement at the level of health care systems, from local office settings to national networks of care. Practitioners of continuous quality improvement integrate knowledge of generalizable scientific evidence with unique clinical practice environments. The following Clinical Improvement Formula provides a model of this concept[13]:

Generalizable Scientific Evidence + Particular Context → Measured Performance Improvement

The formula builds on complex and interdependent systems of knowledge. Indeed, not only the textual elements of this formula but also its syntactic connectors, the "+" and "→" signs, embed specific operational tasks and depend on specific cognitive skills. Figure 1-3, below, illustrates essential forms of knowledge required for successful performance of each step. These steps are described as follows:

- **Generalizable Scientific Evidence.** The essential function here is locating, acquiring, and evaluating biomedical knowledge—that is, the evidence. Practitioners of clinical improvement must be skilled in evidence-based practice techniques of forming answerable questions, retrieving appropriate studies, critically appraising those studies, and

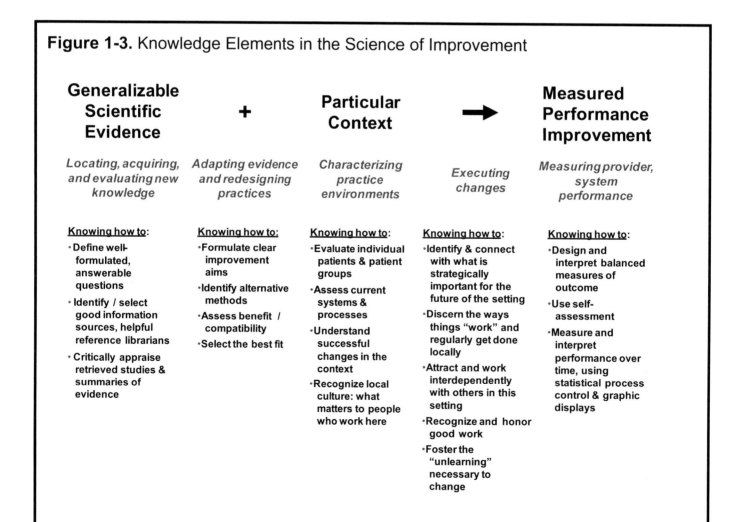

Figure 1-3. Knowledge Elements in the Science of Improvement

Generalizable Scientific Evidence	+	Particular Context	→	Measured Performance Improvement
Locating, acquiring, and evaluating new knowledge	*Adapting evidence and redesigning practices*	*Characterizing practice environments*	*Executing changes*	*Measuring provider, system performance*
Knowing how to: • Define well-formulated, answerable questions • Identify / select good information sources, helpful reference librarians • Critically appraise retrieved studies & summaries of evidence	**Knowing how to:** • Formulate clear improvement aims • Identify alternative methods • Assess benefit / compatibility • Select the best fit	**Knowing how to:** • Evaluate individual patients & patient groups • Assess current systems & processes • Understand successful changes in the context • Recognize local culture: what matters to people who work here	**Knowing how to:** • Identify & connect with what is strategically important for the future of the setting • Discern the ways things "work" and regularly get done locally • Attract and work interdependently with others in this setting • Recognize and honor good work • Foster the "unlearning" necessary to change	**Knowing how to:** • Design and interpret balanced measures of outcome • Use self-assessment • Measure and interpret performance over time, using statistical process control & graphic displays

The essential forms of knowledge required for successful performance of each step of the Clinical Improvement Formula are shown.

interpreting the use of analytic techniques. Many of these studies have tested hypotheses in context-free settings, resulting in knowledge that is insufficient to actualize improvement in real-world clinical settings.

- **The "+" Sign.** The syntactic connector indicates that the acquisition of generalizable scientific evidence is not enough. Knowing the evidence does not ensure that the knowledge will be successfully integrated. The "+" sign serves as a bridging domain of knowledge that supports adapting evidence and redesigning practices. Effective leaders of change know how to assess innovations for compatibility with the current system, how to design and sequence specific care algorithms to match locally available resources, and how to manage conflict and negotiation in the context of unique practice histories.

- **Particular Context.** Practitioners of clinical improvement are adept at characterizing unique practice environments and can interpret data (both quantitative and qualitative) based on local priorities and performance, assess the populations' clinical and demographic characteristics, and evaluate the organizations' structures and interactions. This knowledge system focuses sharply on the particular setting and all that contributes to its identity.

- **The "→" Sign.** After bridging the generalizable scientific evidence and the particular context, expertise is required to support the actual execution of changes. This domain requires skills in effective communication, articulating a vision, supporting staff during change, and embedding strategies for sustainability and long-term development.

- **Measured Performance Improvement.** As described in subsequent chapters, successful improvement over time depends on reliable and recurrent measurement of provider and system performance. Use of statistical process control charts, graphic displays, and other clinical assessment tools provides not only feedback data on improvement trends but also "feed-forward" information to facilitate

point-of-care improvement in real-time practice.

Sustained and meaningful change is grounded in the knowledge systems derived from the Clinical Improvement Formula. The necessary skills can be learned, and (more important) they can also be practiced.

Priority of Clinical Outcomes

Clinicians focus on clinical outcomes. The outcomes most concerning to providers are the heart attacks, strokes, and kidney failure that Mr. Clarke and Mr. Jarvis may have 10 years from now as a result of complications from uncontrolled diabetes. However, without careful attention to such short-term outcomes as physical functioning, mental health, and patient satisfaction, it is unlikely that their providers will achieve their long-term clinical goals. Patient-centered care is important, but its significance lies in the fact that without providing care that meets the needs of patients on their own terms, we are unlikely to help them stay healthy in the long run.

In the cases of Mr. Clarke and Mr. Jarvis, the domains of relevant outcomes are readily apparent. A first domain is clinical: The impact of chronic disease and its treatment on morbidity and mortality are of high importance. What physiological and pathophysiological changes occur as a result of uncontrolled chronic diseases? What benefits and complications are associated with a selected treatment? Functional health status is a second domain of great importance. After surviving their acute symptomatic episodes, can Mr. Clarke and Mr. Jarvis control their chronic diseases and return to their prior employment; participate actively, productively, and happily in community and family life; and reduce their risk of experiencing future acute exacerbations of their chronic illnesses? Satisfaction against need is a third essential outcome domain. How do Mr. Clarke and Mr. Jarvis perceive the quality of care and services they received, and to what extent have their needs and expectations for care been met? Finally, the fourth outcome domain of cost includes both direct health care expenses (incurred in the provision of clinical care) and indirect social costs that arise from lost time at work or nonparticipation in other home-based or community-based affairs (that is, social role activities). Have these costs been minimized as much as possible?

These four cardinal outcome domains of clinical, functional, satisfaction, and cost are unified in the model of a Clinical Value Compass,[14,15] which is discussed in greater detail in Chapter 4. Each outcome domain can be understood, measured, evaluated, and improved using methods that are introduced later in this book. As depicted in Figure 1-4, below, the Clinical Value Compass helps us clarify favorable outcomes in terms of clinical and functional status, satisfaction, and cost. The Clinical Value Compass helps us clarify favorable outcomes in each of the domains, and "value" can be understood as a ratio of improved clinical, functional, and satisfaction outcomes over costs. Using this approach to identify specific and comprehensive measures for each point in

the compass permits us to assess value more precisely. Subsequent chapters of this book analyze components of value in much greater detail and explore means by which all clinicians can participate in sustaining and increasing value.

The Work of Everyone

Because quality improvement is not routinely built into clinical training experiences nor explicitly mandated in most job descriptions, many health care professionals consider such activities to be outside their usual scope of practice and responsibility. Quality improvement thus becomes synonymous with extra effort rather than incorporated into daily work. As a result, improvement tasks are delegated to special quality improvement teams or resentfully squeezed in during administrative or personal time.

But when professionals can reflect on and reframe their implicit assumptions, clinical improvement becomes recognized as a necessary

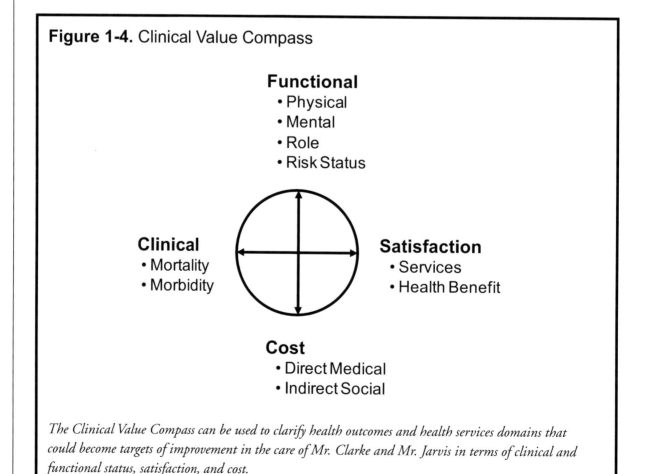

Figure 1-4. Clinical Value Compass

Functional
- Physical
- Mental
- Role
- Risk Status

Clinical
- Mortality
- Morbidity

Satisfaction
- Services
- Health Benefit

Cost
- Direct Medical
- Indirect Social

The Clinical Value Compass can be used to clarify health outcomes and health services domains that could become targets of improvement in the care of Mr. Clarke and Mr. Jarvis in terms of clinical and functional status, satisfaction, and cost.

component of patient care itself. Highly effective clinicians and organizations understand that improving the work is part of the work. Conceived this way, the activities of patient care, practice improvement, and professional learning are interdependent and mutually supportive. As depicted in Figure 1-5, below, quality improvement work is understood more inclusively as "the combined and unceasing efforts of everyone—healthcare professionals, patients and their families, researchers, payers, planners and educators—to make the changes that will lead to better patient outcomes (health), better system performance (care), and better professional development (learning)."[13(p. 2)] The work of quality improvement requires optimal functioning as an interprofessional health care team that includes the patient and his or her family to address such issues as patient motivation and self-efficacy to truly improve the quality of care experienced by the patient.

The work of change and improvement must be understood as an intrinsic part of everyone's job, every day, in all parts of the system. Considering how to improve our work changes our thinking about the "extra" work of quality improvement and can create engagement in thinking about how patients can receive the best care possible.

Figure 1-5. Engaging Everyone in the Clinical Value Compass, Clinical Microsystems, and the Clinical Improvement Formula

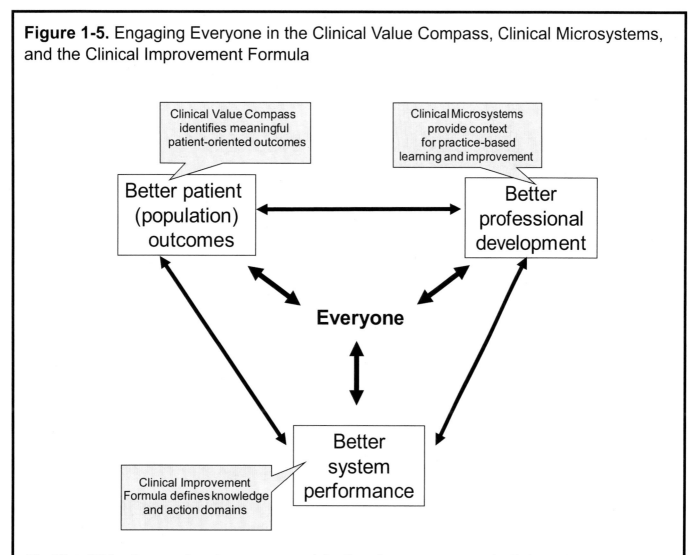

The Clinical Value Compass, clinical microsystems, and the Clinical Improvement Formula all play a role in contributing to better patient outcomes, system performance, and professional development.

Ready to Climb

In assessing the cases of Mr. Clarke and Mr. Jarvis, we begin to recognize the potential impact of the Clinical Value Compass and improvement-oriented thinking, along with knowledge of systems and microsystem organization, on care, as summarized in the following lessons:

- **Clinicians Working in High-Functioning Microsystems Develop Protocols and Pathways to Manage Routine Interventions with Great Efficiency.** Although quality "happens" one patient at a time, these streamlined, efficient processes of care are the primary focus of quality improvement efforts. Consistent delivery of such quality requires both rigorous attention to the latest scientific evidence and specific adaptation to well-understood contexts specific to individual patients, units, and clinics. Available evidence, both general and contextual, must be integrated in real time—that is, during the swift daily flow of patient care—and under circumstances that are often ambiguous. The reflective clinician and the reflective interprofessional team embrace these challenges as continuous learning opportunities.

- **Improvement Is Too Big a Job to Delegate.** Because quality, safety, and efficiency are determined continuously in each clinical encounter, the responsibility for maintaining quality belongs to every member of the health care organization. As we have previously stated, the expectation in clinical settings must be that every participant has two jobs—to *do* the work and to *improve* the work. Such a mandate requires that physicians, nurses, pharmacists, social workers, therapists, administrative personnel, and others throughout the organization receive basic training in quality improvement methods and that all staff be encouraged and expected to use these skills in daily work. Leaders of health care organizations must in turn develop a broad and deep improvement infrastructure (for example, frontline training, informatics, safety climate) to nurture the growth of this quality culture.

- **Quality Measurement and Transparency Will Profoundly Change the Work of Health Care Systems.** Employers, accreditation agencies, regulators, payers, and the public monitor evidence-based metrics.[16,17] The result is that as metrics for both quality and cost (the two components of "value") grow more accurate, pervasive, and transparent, informed patients will selectively entrust their care—and informed purchasers will selectively channel their beneficiaries—to health care organizations that achieve the highest levels of demonstrable quality.

Several decades have passed since sociologist Robert Lynd implored his academic audience to ask of their own scholarly endeavors, "Knowledge for what?"[18] Clinician-scientists of the twenty-first century must ask themselves this same question. What are we trying to achieve in our frontline care of patients and populations, and what forms of knowledge, practice, and continuous learning are necessary to accomplish this goal?

In this chapter we have introduced broad concepts such as the Clinical Value Compass, systems thinking, and the clinical microsystem to guide the learner through the remainder of the book and through the challenging process of incorporating quality improvement into the daily work of our real-world practice settings. The Clinical Value Compass facilitates our understanding of patient-oriented outcomes. Systems thinking and use of the clinical microsystem approach remind us that achievement of these outcomes depends on thoughtful adaptation of scientific evidence to locally defined contexts while coordinating care among interprofessional team members. This process of adaptation and implementation is the daily work of frontline clinical microsystems, which serve as both the supportive context and the substrate for practice-based learning and professional development. Success depends on both individual and collective, interprofessional competence in multiple domains of knowledge and skill.

Because several of these domains fall outside the usual training of physicians, nurses, and other health care professionals, we are all on the steep slope of our learning curve in our clinical practice. This is an exciting place to be, so long as we embrace our roles as continuous learners. In the chapters that follow, we begin our climb up this learning curve. Through specific exercises and case studies, we bring clinical improvement and practice-based learning into the daily work of patient care, with the goal of optimizing that care continuously in our own practice settings.

References

1. Applewhite A, Evans WR III, Frothingham A. *And I Quote: The Definitive Collection of Quotes, Sayings, and Jokes for the Contemporary Speechmaker,* rev. ed. New York: St. Martin's Press, 2003.

2. Brennan TA, et al. Incidence of adverse events and negligence in hospitalized patients. Results of the Harvard Medical Practice Study I. *N Engl J Med.* 1991 Feb 7;324(6):370–376.

3. Leape LL, et al. The nature of adverse events in hospitalized patients. Results of the Harvard Medical Practice Study II. *N Engl J Med.* 1991 Feb 7;324(6):377–384.

4. Kohn LT, Corrigan JM, Donaldson MS; Committee on Quality of Health Care in America. *To Err Is Human: Building a Safer Health System.* Washington, DC: National Academy Press, 2000.

5. Commonwealth Fund. Public Reporting and Transparency. Commonwealth Fund pub. no. 988. Colmers J. Jan 2007. Accessed Oct 14, 2012. http://www.commonwealthfund.org/~/media/Files/Publications/Fund%20Report/2007/Feb/Public%20Reporting%20and%20Transparency/Colmers_pubreportingtransparency_988%20pdf.pdf.

6. US Department of Health & Human Services. Hospital Compare. (Updated: Oct 11, 2012.) Accessed Oct 14, 2012. http://www.hospitalcompare.hhs.gov.

7. Milstein A. Ending extra payment for "never events"— Stronger incentives for patients' safety. *N Engl J Med.* 2009 Jun 4;360(23):2388–2390.

8. Centers for Medicare & Medicaid Services. Medicare and Medicaid programs: Hospital outpatient prospective payment; ambulatory surgical center payment; hospital value-based purchasing program; physician self-referral; and patient notification requirements in provider agreements. Final rule with comment period. *Fed Regist.* 2011 Nov 30;76(230):74122–74584.

9. Zigmond J. Innovation won't wait: Despite law's uncertainty, CMS awards grants. *Mod Healthc.* 2012 May 14;42(20):12.

10. National Health Service Institute for Innovation and Improvement. Annual Report and Accounts of the NHS Institute for Innovation and Improvement 2010–11. 2011. Accessed Oct 14, 2012. http://www.institute.nhs.uk/images/documents/NHS%20Institute%20Annual%20Report%20and%20Accounts%202010-11%2012%20July%202011.pdf.

11. Nelson EC, Batalden PB, Godfrey MM, editors. *Quality by Design: A Clinical Microsystems Approach.* San Francisco: Jossey-Bass, 2007.

12. Reason J. *Managing the Risks of Organization Accidents.* Burlington, VT: Ashgate, 1997.

13. Batalden PB, Davidoff F. What is "quality improvement" and how can it transform healthcare? *Qual Saf Health Care.* 2007 Feb;16(1):2–3.

14. Nelson EC, et al. Improving health care, Part 2: A clinical improvement worksheet and users' manual. *Jt Comm J Qual Improv.* 1996 Aug;22(8):531–548.

15. Nelson EC, et al. Improving health care, Part 1: The Clinical Value Compass. *Jt Comm J Qual Improv.* 1996 Apr;22(4):243–258.

16. Committee on Redesigning Health Insurance Performance Measures, Payment, and Performance Improvement Programs, Institute of Medicine. *Performance Measurement: Accelerating Improvement.* Washington, DC: National Academies Press, 2006.

17. National Quality Forum (MQF). *National Priorities for Healthcare Quality Measurement and Reporting: A Consensus Report.* Washington, DC: NQF, 2004.

18. Lynd RS. *Knowledge for What? The Place of Social Science in American Culture.* Princeton, NJ: Princeton University Press, 1939.

Chapter 2

Getting Started and Identifying Targets for Change

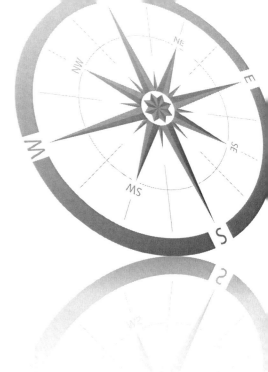

David E. Willens, Lorraine C. Mion, Eugene C. Nelson, Paul B. Batalden, Robert S. Dittus

Quality is never an accident. It is always the result of intelligent effort. There must be the will to produce a superior thing.
—John Ruskin (1819–1900)[1]

Most health professionals understand that clinical systems, large and small, are in need of improvement. Knowing how to initiate this improvement in local practice settings is less intuitive. Initiating change presents various challenges, including finding time for improvement, learning how to plan and execute a project, and identifying targets for change that are both meaningful and achievable.[2,3] Additional challenges arise in implementing changes that have been requested from levels of institutional leadership perceived as removed from the local practice setting. Whether the desire or target for change is initiated from the "ground up" or the "top down," establishing the motivation to change and getting the team on board are essential. This chapter explores these challenges to getting started. The steps that follow can be tailored to the specific needs and constraints of individual clinical settings, but the general framework has broad applicability across practice settings.

The Challenges of Getting Started

Just getting started can pose a challenge—several challenges, in fact. These challenges include time, know-how, and where to start.

Challenge 1: Time

Often, lack of time is cited as a barrier to initiating work-related improvements. Everyone is busy, and the best people for the job are often the busiest. But everyone has the same amount of time in a day; people just choose to segment it differently on the basis of personal and professional values. When time is noted to be unavailable for improvement work, such a perception can result from a tacit belief that improvement is not part of regular work (as discussed in Chapter 1). By acknowledging that "work" and "work improvement" are synonymous and recognizing the efficiency that emerges from ongoing quality innovation, the busy professional integrates regular improvement time into work routines. This integration can be achieved, for example, by holding daily team huddles (of brief duration) during which clinical operations are discussed and small changes to clinical work are planned. In this manner, frontline operations and continuous improvements become increasingly indistinguishable.

In addition, many people mistake activity for accomplishment. Being busy does not guarantee productivity and sometimes undermines it. Valuable time can often be created for improvement projects by eliminating busywork or unnecessary activity. Eliminating common time-wasting activity can enhance productivity, efficiency, quality, and satisfaction at work.

Challenge 2: Know-How

Institutional, team, and individual commitment and dedicated time are necessary for any improvement process, and specific know-how (made up of knowledge, attitudes, skills, and behaviors) is essential. As shown in the chapters that follow, such know-how can be acquired through learning about and applying the practice-based clinical improvement strategies. But mastery of the entire canon of quality improvement techniques is not required to get started. Some general knowledge and skills can be easily learned and applied creatively in both personal and professional domains.

"Students" of quality improvement—including practicing clinicians—should develop personal improvement projects early in their own process of practice-based learning. This experience enables individuals to "see" with different eyes, to appreciate that anything can be improved with direct attention. In addition, many of the principles and methods employed in clinical improvement work are similarly applicable in personal contexts, and recognition of this overlap can serve as a valuable bridge to mastery with more formal methods.

For example, in some quality improvement courses, students identify a personal goal, such as regular exercise, daily practice with a musical instrument or sport, or keeping up with e-mail correspondence.[4,5] This goal becomes the focus of a personal improvement initiative for which implementation includes defining specific targets, anticipating potential barriers, developing detailed plans, recording observations on progress toward the goal, and reflecting on outcomes. This extended exercise is based on a model developed by Roberts and Sergesketter in a classic book, *Quality Is Personal: A Foundation for Total Quality Management.*[6] It reveals to students the extent to which challenges to continuous improvement (clinical or otherwise) can be anticipated and overcome.

Too often, quality improvement techniques are presented as a set of statistical and group process tools that will magically create improvement by themselves. When this improvement does not happen, the tools might be prematurely dismissed as ineffective and the motivation for improvement dismissed as ill conceived. The matching of personally and professionally meaningful improvement targets with well-chosen methods will increase the likelihood of success.

Challenge 3: Where to Start

Many practitioners remain unsure of how to identify targets for clinical improvement. Even when individuals and teams are committed to quality and familiar with improvement principles and techniques, they may be unsure where to focus their energy and resources. A common question is, "How do we find things to improve?" Sometimes senior or midlevel management establishes improvement targets, and sometimes frontline individuals and teams identify targets for change based on their intimate knowledge of daily work. Finding the intersection between each of these perspectives is often a fruitful area in which to start.

Organizations have strategic priorities. Because financial, time, and human resources are limited, each organization must choose areas on which to focus. Activities in health care are usually prioritized in areas such as people, service, growth, finance, and, more recently, quality. The strategic priorities are often general statements such as "Elevate employee satisfaction"; "Expand referring physician base"; or "Achieve lowest mortality rate." These are broad goals that guide the specific projects within almost every department from accounting to environmental services to nursing. Measures for these specific projects, such as rates of aspirin use in patients admitted with heart attacks, as well as aggregate metrics that track the success of more global initiatives, such as mortality rates, are often followed electronically on "dashboards" that are accessible to those within the organization.[6] Improvement activities that support these priorities are more likely to receive attention and resources from leadership. Indeed, leadership priority setting is a core quality improvement capability and often determines dashboards for the organization.[7]

How these priority areas for action are addressed is often up to each department or practice area. Ideas for improvements that originate locally are often the most successful. Local leadership commonly plans and then delegates these projects, but often the most realistic and achievable ideas for accomplishing improvements come from workers at the front line who understand what might work and why. Changing work flow and behavior is difficult; people are more likely to become engaged in a project or excited about a change into which they have input.

Quality improvement or accreditation/regulation compliance departments can also be a source for improvement ideas. Health care systems are required to track and report rates of many outcome measures of clinical processes, such as catheter-related bloodstream infections, patient falls, and chronic disease monitoring to organizations such as the Centers for Medicare & Medicaid Services (CMS) and The Joint Commission. Often teams of individuals in departments of quality and compliance are dedicated to the collection of these data. These departments can sometimes help with coaching a project team, granting access to electronic medical record information, or analyzing data.

Support from an organization's top leaders is vital to nurture and sustain practice-based learning and improvement efforts, but some degree of improvement work is possible even in organizational cultures that lack systemwide support. Everyone can create a climate of learning and improvement in their own workplace that makes positive change not only possible but also regularly achievable. Opportunity almost always exists for frontline workers, using their expertise of local processes, work flow, or patient care, to initiate small improvements in their work environments. The following section will assist in identifying targets for change within a health care system.

Identifying Targets for Improvement in Clinical Care

The goal of clinical improvement is better health care system performance reflected in better patient outcomes. The successful achievement of this goal requires effort and collaboration of numerous individuals, from administrators to frontline workers, from professionals to unlicensed personnel. Thus, opportunities for improvement exist everywhere and in every facet of clinical care.

The first step in clinical improvement, identifying the target for improvement, can be accomplished at the organizational level or at the practitioner's level. The 12 action probes that follow provide the practitioner and midlevel administrator with practical approaches in identifying targets. They can be done singly or in combination to generate multiple improvement ideas. For professionals already committed to specific quality concerns, this same exercise can focus the improvement efforts or broaden the scope of contexts in which specific strategies are applied.

Action Probe 1: Talk to Insiders— Ask the Staff

Most clinical practices cannot afford the luxury of an external consulting group to identify potential improvement areas. In fact, all health care settings are rich with internal experts: clinicians, nurses, receptionists, administrators, and many others who experience the problems of service delivery every day. Indeed, staff members are among the best-informed consultants.

To obtain the benefit of their considerable expertise and insights, ask any five people in the relevant staff groups that follow to complete the following two statements. You might use e-mail, but brief in-person discussions can reveal much more.

1. The "clinical work" that needs to be improved if we want better patient outcomes (or specify the desired quality improvement) is

   _____.

2. The reason(s) the system's performance is not as good as it could be is (are)

   _____.

   Here is a list of staff to approach:
   - New employees
   - Employees who are getting ready to work elsewhere
   - Information desk staff and receptionists

- Volunteer workers
- Administrative assistants, managers, officers
- Quality, utilization review, and risk management staff
- Finance, purchasing, and billing office staff
- Scheduling staff
- Physician providers (including medical students, residents, fellows, moonlighters)
- Physician assistants
- Nurses (including advanced practice nurses, nurse practitioners)
- Pharmacists
- Social workers
- Clinical therapists (physical, occupational, respiratory, among others)

Action Probe 2: Engage the Beneficiaries of Clinical Care—Ask Patients, Their Families, and Other Stakeholders

The direct and indirect beneficiaries of health care services have strong feelings about the quality (or safety) of care (both the way it is provided and the outcomes of care). Research shows that patients and their families are able to identify and communicate safety and quality concerns to their providers.[8] Programs to engage patients have become popular in many health care systems. They encourage patients to speak up by asking questions or pointing out potential problems in their care (such as hand washing). Some patients are too sick to participate, and providers must not shift the responsibility for safety toward patients, families, or others. They can, however, add new perspectives in identifying opportunities to improve care.[3]

Approach individuals on the following list:
- Patients
- Family members
- Employers (who benefit from healthy employees and who pay for care)
- Purchasers (who pay for care or administer claims)
- Staff of other health care facilities (long term care, rehabilitation centers, and others)

Ask any five people in the relevant groups to complete the following four statements about the health care they receive; a brief in-person discussion is usually fruitful.

1. This practice (clinic, unit, etc.) could improve _____ services to lessen the burden of illness for its patients.
2. This practice (clinic, unit, etc.) could improve the way it delivers care and make patients' lives easier or better by _____.
3. The things that I hear people complaining about in this practice (clinic, unit, etc.) include _____.
4. It costs me _____ to use this practice.

Action Probe 3: Explore the Literature— What Have Others Done?

A growing number of public resources can facilitate identification of evidence-based guidelines and practice-based best practices for high-quality clinical care, including the following sources:

- National Guideline Clearinghouse—a joint effort of the Agency for Healthcare Research and Quality (AHRQ), the American Association of Health Plans (now called America's Health Insurance Plans), and the American Medical Association—which provides full text and abstracts of clinical practice (http://www.guideline.gov)
- Institute for Clinical Systems Improvement (http://www.icsi.org)
- Specialty Societies (for example, American College of Physicians Quality Improvement Programs: http://www.acponline.org/running_practice/quality_improvement)
- Institute for Healthcare Improvement (http://www.ihi.org)
- Agency for Healthcare Research and Quality (http://www.ahrq.gov), including AHRQ Health Care Innovations Exchange and AHRQ Patient Safety Network
- CMS Quality Initiatives (http://www.cms.gov/QualityInitiativesGenInfo)
- Networking with colleagues working in clinical improvement through professional societies such as the Academy for Healthcare Improvement (http://www.a4hi.org)
- Annual meetings of professional societies

Specialist providers will be familiar with other guideline and protocol resources pertinent to particular clinical conditions. Review websites of organizations that promote quality and safety of health care.

For designated targets of improvement, a search of the health services and health care literature using key terms will also yield programs, reports, and research conducted in the area. A professional journal such as *The Joint Commission Journal on Quality and Patient Safety* makes a particularly good starting point. The AHRQ Patient Safety Network provides the latest annotated links to patient safety literature.

Action Probe 4: Look at What Others Know About Local Practice— From the Outside Looking In

Performance transparency is increasingly required in health care systems. Clinical work is now monitored, quantified, and compared to external standards. (*See* Chapters 4 and 5 for further discussion.) Practitioners can gain valuable insight from data that have been externally collected on their own health care practices. For instance, CMS posts comparative reports for hospitals, nursing homes, and practitioners (http://www.hospitalcompare.hhs.gov). Improvement teams can learn from competitors who have attracted patients by providing greater value in specific contexts. Consider any clinical service in which your organization or service is not the region's leading high-quality, low-cost provider and evaluate why the competitor is doing better. In addition, many organizations offer certifications or standardized solutions for implementing best practices.

Review comparative results or best-practice quality improvement programs from the following sources:
- Joint Commission survey results and performance data (http://www.healthcarequalitydata.org/)
- CMS Resource Locator (http://www.medicare.gov/help-and-resources/find-doctors-hospitals-and-facilities/quality-care-finder.html)

- Dartmouth Atlas of Health Care (http://www.dartmouthatlas.org)
- National Committee for Quality Assurance surveys and Healthcare Effectiveness Data and Information Set (HEDIS) results (http://www.ncqa.org)
- Statewide databases on charges, costs, utilization, and outcomes

Action Probe 5: Treasure the Failures— If It's Broken, Fix It

Failures refer to malfunctions, near misses (also called *close calls*), or errors of omission or commission. In the majority of cases, these events are not the fault of a single person but instead are indicators of a systemic process in need of improvement.[9] Because an important goal is to reduce the frequency and negative impact of such events, failures must paradoxically be embraced— that is, recognized, measured, fixed, and examined for lessons learned that could be applicable to other situations.

Health care systems now routinely track many events that could each signal broader safety or quality problems. The following manifestations of failures may indicate areas in need of improvement:
- Risk management claims made (and cost)
- Complaints made by patients and families
- Medical error reports
- Adverse event reports
- Incident reports
- Quality improvement department reports
- Internal audit reports
- Near-miss reports

Action Probe 6: Review Customer and Other Stakeholder Survey Results

Every organization performs satisfaction or perception-of-care surveys, and the resulting data can stimulate multiple improvement ideas. Review surveys completed by the following:
- Patients and families
- Employees
- Medical staff
- Community residents
- Referring physicians

Action Probe 7: Understand the Current Process

Clinical processes, such as patient check-in or medical procedures, connect team members to patients and to one another and are rich with opportunities for improvement. Identify and map a current ("as is") step-by-step process of care (from both staff and patient perspectives): Follow pathways of information flow, observe clinical steps, talk to people (patients, providers, support staff) about how things really work at the front line, and search for recurrent problems. Do not map the ideal or intended process—map the real process!

In reality, one or more of the following process challenges identified might be an important target for improvement work:
- Bottlenecks, waits, delays, queuing
- Interruptions
- Communication failures
- Equipment failures
- Errors and near misses
- Misplaced charts, equipment, or other necessary tools
- Steps that require exceptional effort to be performed properly
- Steps that involve multiple decisions
- Frustrations, irritations, and anger
- Work-arounds, rework, and "do-overs"

Action Probe 8: Walk in Their Shoes— Play the Role

Most health care workers can recall their own frustrations as recipients of health care services. Participant observation can identify numerous steps in clinical encounters that patients might experience as frustrating; these are obvious targets for ongoing improvement. Play the role of patient, or of another professional, and walk through the following steps:
- Being admitted
- Visiting a clinician
- Calling the clinician's office
- Being "handed off" to another provider (nurse or physician) or another unit
- Using an outpatient service
- Going to the emergency department
- Being discharged home or to another facility

Action Probe 9: Review Internal Data

Health care organizations generate mountains of data. As another way to identify frequently performed activities, using internal reports, identify the practice's or clinical program's top 10 conditions in terms of any (or all) of the following parameters:
- Volume
- Costs
- Charges
- Amount of time spent
- Risk to patient
- Achievable benefit not achieved (ABNA—that is, the gap between what is thought to be possible and what is currently happening)

Action Probe 10: Identify "Sinkholes" of Temporary Help

Although periodic shifts in work flow and other labor market forces might necessitate occasional hiring of temporary help (including float staff), the regular use of such workers can be costly, inefficient, and labor intensive (for staff who must oversee training) and might increase the risk of clinical or administrative errors.

Find the locations where temporary workers, or "temps," are hired most frequently. Identify whether work redesign can avoid the need for temps; if not, standardize work to minimize the risk of errors being generated by temps.

Action Probe 11: Eliminate Waste— Look for Muda

Muda is a Japanese term that reflects the concept of shame arising from waste—wasted time, wasted effort, and wasted resources. (*See* Sidebar 2-1 on page 19 for details.)

To find waste and to eliminate it, ask the same five people who served as insider problem spotters to complete the following three statements:
1. One thing we do all the time that accomplishes very little is _____.
2. In my area, we always have plenty of _____, because only _____ ever uses them.
3. In my area, we could save money by _____.

Sidebar 2-1. What Is *Muda*?

The Japanese word *muda* translates, roughly, to the concept of "futility and uselessness." Taichi Ohno, who led Toyota Motor Company's quality efforts for many years, used the term to signify activity without value, and in this sense *muda* can be found almost anywhere in our personal lives and organizational work. Our interpretation here is built on insights from Ohno, Harry V. Roberts, Bernard F. Sergesketter, and others.

Muda of resource consumption is the use of work and supplies that consume time or money without adding value. For example, *muda* is present when we ask patients repeatedly for the same identifying and demographic information. In administrative work, we experience *muda* when starting meetings late, not sticking to an agenda, or attending meetings at which our presence is not needed.

Muda of inventory is buildup of inventories (of services or products) that no one wants. In health care, an example of this buildup is unused hospital beds.

Muda of action is the presence of unnecessary process steps. In health care, *muda* of action (that is, action without the need for action) can be found in excessive testing, in convoluted scheduling rules, in reports that no one uses, and in continuous monitoring of noncritical patients.

Muda of transport is the movement of people, equipment, or information without purpose. Examples in health care include movement of patients from labor to delivery to recovery rooms and multiple trips to the supply cart.

Muda of waiting occurs downstream when people or processes upstream are late. An example in health care is surgery delay or cancellation because lab reports are unavailable.

Muda in meeting stakeholder needs includes services or products that do not match priorities of patients or other beneficiaries. Patients are all too familiar with education materials that fail to answer their practical questions, with medications not taken, and with hearing aids that stay in drawers.

Reference

Roberts HV, Sergesketter BF. *Quality Is Personal: A Foundation for Total Quality Management*. New York: Free Press, 1993.

Ask the same five people identified earlier to complete the following two statements:

1. At _____ (institution), we always have to wait for_____ _____.

2. At _____ (institution), we really need or greatly prefer _____, but we usually or often get _____.

Action Probe 12: Probe the Process More Deeply—Use Change Concepts

Change concepts (described further in Chapter 6) are general high-leverage ideas that stimulate creative problem solving and promote novel ways of thinking—including generation of specific improvement strategies.[2,10,11]

Identify an important clinical service (using one of the previously described action probes) and apply one of the following change concepts:

- Modify input.
- Combine steps.
- Eliminate failures at transitions.
- Eliminate a step.
- Reorder the sequence of steps.
- Change an element in the process by creating an arrangement with another party who can perform the step more efficiently.
- Replace a step with an alternative that has better value.
- Redesign production on the basis of knowledge of the service or product that is created.
- Redesign the service or product on the basis of knowledge of use of the service or product.
- Redesign the process with knowledge of need and aim.

Narrowing the List and Moving Forward

Those who participate in the process of generating improvement ideas will identify more ideas for positive change than can be implemented with available time and resources. An important next step is to prioritize the improvement ideas from the generated list using explicit criteria, such as those that will have the greatest impact or those that are the most feasible to implement. *Impact* would include such domains as the potential improvements in quality of patient care, reductions in cost, and critical interest among important stakeholders. *Feasibility* would include such domains as the time, resources, and skills needed to test the idea. Narrowing of the list can be accomplished in multiple ways. One common approach is to use a process called *multivoting*,[2,12] in which each team member votes for his or her top 25% choices of improvement ideas. The votes of all team members are tabulated and then ranked in the order of most to least votes received. Additional rounds can follow until a clear preference is established. Because individuals will likely use the impact and feasibility priority criteria differently in performing these rankings, if the organization or its leadership has a clear preference for the relative importance of these priority criteria, this aspect should be discussed prior to voting.

In summary, by confronting initial challenges to change and by exploring local sources of information already available to most clinical practices (including staff and patient expertise, internal and external collections of data, and reflective assessment of process dynamics), a large list of specific improvement ideas can be generated. From this list a smaller set of the most achievable ideas can be defined. With this list in hand, specific improvement strategies can be developed that will improve clinical value through attention to identified targets. In the next chapter, to support development of these strategies, the Clinical Improvement Worksheet is introduced. It is a powerful tool that facilitates translation of improvement ideas into specific action plans.

References

1. Goodreads. John Ruskin Quotes. Ruskin J. Accessed Nov 26, 2012. http://www.goodreads.com/author/quotes/1606.John_Ruskin?page=2.

2. Nelson EC, Batalden PB, Godfrey MM, editors. *Quality by Design: A Clinical Microsystems Approach.* San Francisco: Jossey-Bass, 2007.

3. Nelson EC, et al., editors. *Value by Design: Developing Clinical Microsystems to Achieve Organizational Excellence.* San Francisco: Jossey-Bass, 2011.

4. Kyrkjebø JM, Hanestad BR. Personal improvement project in nursing education: Learning methods and tools for continuous quality improvement in nursing practice. *J Adv Nurs.* 2003 Jan;41(1):88–98.

5. Neuhauser D. Personal continuous quality improvement workbook. Accessed Oct 26, 2012. http://www.a4hi.org/docs/Neuhauser_personal_improvement_project_workbook.pdf.

6. Roberts HV, Sergesketter BF. *Quality Is Personal: A Foundation for Total Quality Management.* New York: Free Press, 1993.

7. Schilling L, et al. Kaiser Permanente's performance improvement system, Part 1: From benchmarking to executing on strategic priorities. *Jt Comm J Qual Patient Saf.* 2010 Nov;36(11):484–498.

8. Weingart SN. Engaging patients in patient safety. In Berman S, editor: *From Office to Front Line: Essential Issues for Health Care Leaders,* 2nd ed. Oak Brook, IL: Joint Commission Resources, 2012, 109–126.

9. Wu AW, ed. *The Value of Close Calls in Improving Patient Safety: Learning How to Avoid and Mitigate Patient Harm.* Oak Brook, IL: Joint Commission Resources, 2011.

10. Langley GJ, Nolan KM, Nolan TW. The foundation of improvement. *Quality Progress.* 1994 Jun;27(6):81–86.

11. de Bono E. *Serious Creativity: Using the Power of Lateral Thinking to Create New Ideas.* New York: HarperBusiness, 1992.

12. Scholtes PR, Joiner BL, Streibel BJ. *The Team Handbook,* 3rd ed. Madison, WI: Oriel, 2003.

Chapter 3

Improving Clinical Care: A Clinical Improvement Worksheet

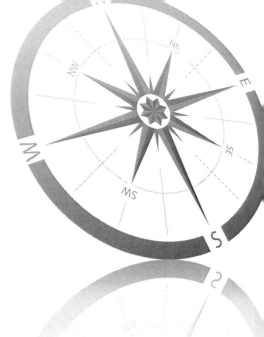

Jennifer D. Thull-Freedman, Rory F. McQuillan, Alene A. Toulany,
Kieran P. McIntyre, Eugene C. Nelson, Paul B. Batalden,
Julie K. Johnson, Joel S. Lazar, Chaim M. Bell

Every system is perfectly designed to get the results it gets.[1(p. 32)]
—Saying popularized by Paul Batalden

Improvement in clinical microsystems proceeds in a manner analogous to patient care itself; both endeavors build on cycles of goal clarification, assessment, intervention, and reassessment. Reflective practitioners of clinical improvement set their aim on specific targets in the caregiving process, clarify these processes through careful analysis, and implement measurable tests of change. Monitoring the outcomes of these interventions permits further refinement of initial goals and of the interventions themselves. Small tests of change can be conducted in everyday clinical practice, enabling individual providers and entire health care teams to learn from and to improve on their work.

In this chapter, we introduce the Clinical Improvement Worksheet, a practical and flexible tool that supports the improvement of patient care in real-world settings. After defining and analyzing a core clinical process in some detail, we review specific steps in the redesign of this process and discuss strategies for testing the impact of redesign on both quality and costs. We examine the improvement worksheet's facilitation of practice-based learning and improvement in a detailed case study, and then we conclude with some general observations on the process of change itself.

The Core Clinical Process

Every episode of care begins with identification of a patient need, continues for short or long durations of time, and might involve multiple patient–clinician encounters in either ambulatory or inpatient settings (or both). Close attention to the structure of these clinical encounters enables us to target specific processes for practice-based improvement.

Each care-seeking episode has three phases: before, during, and after. In most cases, the process begins when a community-dwelling person experiences a new need for health care services such as diagnosis, prevention, treatment, or rehabilitation. Before initiating the care-seeking episode itself, this individual already has a clinical (or biologic) and a functional status, both of which can be assessed and monitored over time. The care seeker also has expectations to be satisfied and a history of costs associated with this particular clinical need. For example, most people have expectations about the way care should be delivered and a set of desired, or "hoped for," health outcomes on the basis of their symptoms and own prior experience or the experience of others. In addition, people incur both direct and indirect costs that are related to the needs that bring them in for care. Over a lifetime, these costs accumulate and create a longitudinal cost profile that derives from accumulated experiences and utilization of health care resources (*see also* discussions of the Clinical Value Compass in Chapters 1 and 4, pages 8 and 38–42).

When a health need is sufficiently compelling, it commonly prompts an individual to access the health care delivery system. On entry into this system, the individual becomes a participant in the core clinical process and a beneficiary of services that clinicians and clinical team members provide. These services can be characterized by the following specific activities:

- Patient assessment, on the basis of data collection from history taking, physical examination, and diagnostic tests
- Diagnosis and classification of the patient's need, on the basis of integration of pertinent information from the aforementioned assessment

- Treatment regimen, determined on the basis of clinical diagnosis and individualized to specific preferences and priorities of the patient
- Follow-up monitoring of the patient and patient's needs over time

The quality and costs of care can be analyzed in terms of the impact of that care on clinical status, functional status, well-being, satisfaction, and costs. The practitioner's challenge is to take action so that each patient experiences the most favorable health outcomes in the most satisfying and least costly manner. The case example in Sidebar 3-1 below illustrates the core clinical process involved in the transition from pediatric to adult kidney transplant care.

The Clinical Improvement Worksheet

How can the improvement of clinical work be incorporated into busy office and hospital routines

---

Sidebar 3-1. Case Example: The Core Clinical Process—Transition to Adult Renal Care

Amber is a 17-year-old student with end-stage kidney disease secondary to chronic kidney disease of unknown etiology (focal and segmental glomerulosclerosis [FSGS]) since the age of 12 years. She received a kidney transplant from her mother at 15 years of age after undergoing peritoneal dialysis for three years. Amber is followed regularly in the pediatric renal transplant clinic and has excellent renal graft function. In late August, just prior to her 18th birthday, her pediatric nephrologist of the last six years tells her that he is transferring her care to a colleague in an adult care hospital. Amber appears unperturbed by the prospect of leaving the pediatric hospital. Although her parents accept this change as inevitable, they express concern about a new team taking over their daughter's care and her ability to navigate the adult health care system.

In September Amber moves into residence at a university campus, where she is studying to be a veterinary assistant. A letter is sent to her family home with information about her first appointment with the adult nephrologist scheduled for early November. Amber's mother calls her to inform her of the clinic appointment. Amber does not attend the appointment, nor does she call the hospital to reschedule. Her mother becomes frustrated and upset about this and calls the hospital. The clinic nurse tells her that Amber needs to contact them directly to reschedule her appointment. Amber calls soon after and is given an appointment a week later,

which she attends. Her blood tests show that although she has stable kidney function, her immunosuppressant-drug levels are low. The transplant coordinator makes several attempts to contact Amber on her cell phone and leaves numerous messages. Amber finally returns the call one week later. The coordinator arranges for her to have repeat drug levels taken in a local hospital. Amber fails to attend this appointment because the time for it conflicts with her examinations. Three weeks later, the renal transplant physician receives a call from another hospital informing him that Amber has been admitted to the local community hospital with a one-week history of fatigue and nausea. Her blood tests are consistent with acute renal failure. She is transferred immediately to the renal transplant center, where she undergoes a kidney biopsy, which shows acute rejection consistent with poor adherence to her medications. Amber undergoes emergent treatment for rejection (plasmapheresis and corticosteroids). Her renal function does not recover and she requires intermittent hemodialysis. Because of the constraints of the hemodialysis schedule, Amber is unable to continue her classes at the university.

On reflection of Amber's case, her transplant physician contemplates that a change to the process of transferring from pediatric to adult care could result in better outcomes for adolescent Amber and other kidney transplant recipients.

---

without disrupting the smooth delivery of care? And how can this improvement be promoted in a manner that builds on clinicians' professional values of science and healing, their intrinsic curiosity about cause and effect, and their personal desire to find the best way to care for their patients?

The Clinical Improvement Worksheet, shown in Figure 3-1 (pages 24–25), is a simple tool designed to facilitate frontline practitioners' blending of clinical improvement work with core processes of actual patient care. Based on a sequential model of quality innovation,[2] the improvement worksheet guides providers through self-assessment of caregiving processes, facilitates application of local knowledge in the development of small tests of change, and directs attention to measures of both health outcomes and cost reduction.

Side A of the worksheet blends improvement thinking with the core clinical process in a manner that practitioners can easily tailor to their own patient care routines. Side B invites more focused attention to the development and implementation of specific tests of change in clinical settings. This graphic, flexible tool offers practitioners a simple format to visualize clinical and improvement processes, to record progress, and to share work in a standardized manner.

In the section that follows, we walk through the Clinical Improvement Worksheet and thus through the generic steps of practice-based improvement work itself. We then demonstrate the improvement worksheet's utility in one application, and we invite readers to experiment with their own local applications. In Appendix A (Figure A-5, pages 143–144) we provide another version, the Improvement Project Worksheet—a "forest view" of the complete improvement process, which helps teams understand the full scope of the project.

Team Up

Improvement efforts benefit from the active engagement of multiple clinical and nonclinical staff. When a collective approach is felt to be most appropriate, core participants must consider early in the endeavor who has greatest knowledge of the clinical process and who should be invited to join the improvement team. This team might

be a natural work group of people who practice together on a daily basis, such as a primary care or obstetrical team, or it might be an ad hoc group brought together to improve management of a specific clinical concern, such as urinary tract infection or total joint replacement. Realistically, not all team members can be selected until specific target populations are identified and until the broad aim of an improvement project is clarified. As the improvement team is developed, the following guidelines should be considered:

- Select individuals who are familiar with various elements of the core process.
- Select individuals from a number of disciplines to reflect diverse areas of expertise and knowledge.
- Designate a leader who is credible and will be actively involved; the leader may be the individual who is responsible for the technical process that needs improvement.
- Limit the number of members to eight or fewer.
- Choose an experienced team facilitator if participants are new to the improvement process.
- If applicable, consider gaining support from institutional management.[3]

Ready . . . Aim . . .

Side A of the Clinical Improvement Worksheet (Figure 3-1, page 24) poses four questions pertinent to the core clinical process and to its ongoing improvement:

Step 1. *Outcomes:* What is the general aim of this work, and who are we trying to help?

Step 2. *Process:* What is the process for giving care to this type of patient?

Step 3. *Changes:* What ideas do we have for changing what is done (the process) to get better results?

Step 4. *Pilot:* How can we pilot test an improvement idea?

Working through Side A provides a high-level view of the core clinical process, directing participants to get ready for change in general and

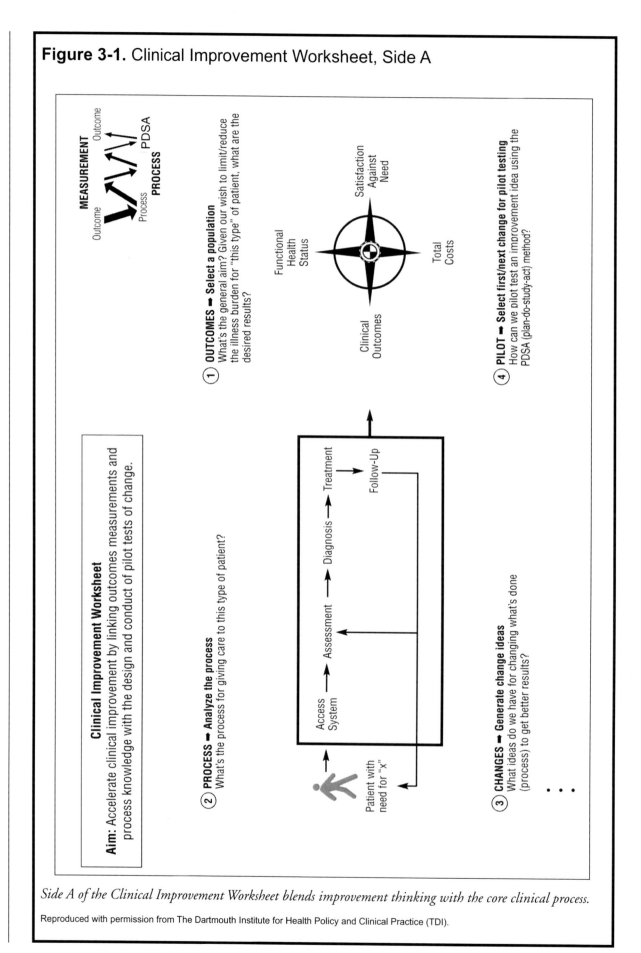

Figure 3-1. Clinical Improvement Worksheet, Side A

Side A of the Clinical Improvement Worksheet blends improvement thinking with the core clinical process.

Reproduced with permission from The Dartmouth Institute for Health Policy and Clinical Practice (TDI).

Figure 3-1. Clinical Improvement Worksheet, Side B

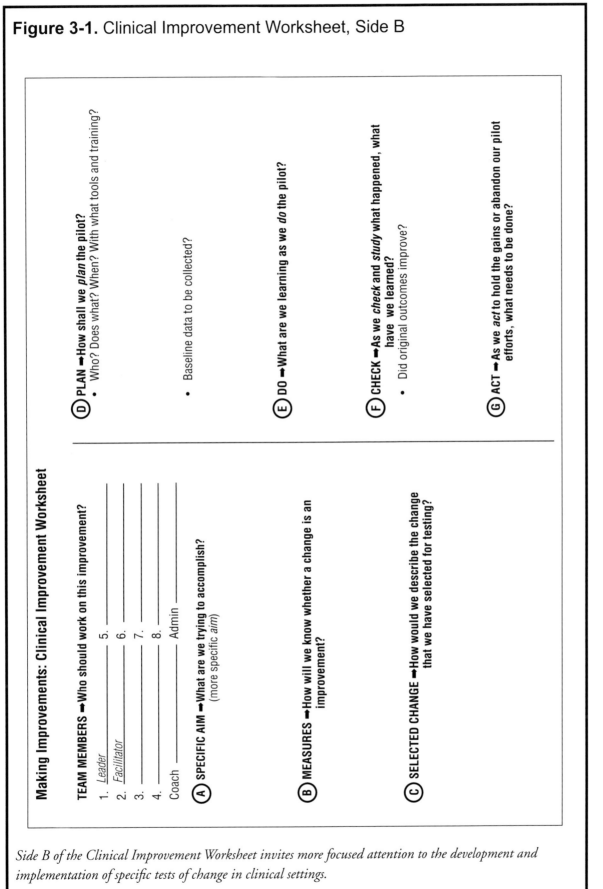

Making Improvements: Clinical Improvement Worksheet

TEAM MEMBERS →Who should work on this improvement?

1. *Leader*　　　5. _____
2. *Facilitator*　　6. _____
3. _____　　　7. _____
4. _____　　　8. _____

Coach _____　　Admin _____

Ⓐ **SPECIFIC AIM →What are we trying to accomplish?**
(more specific *aim*)

Ⓑ **MEASURES →How will we know whether a change is an improvement?**

Ⓒ **SELECTED CHANGE →How would we describe the change that we have selected for testing?**

Ⓓ **PLAN →How shall we *plan* the pilot?**
• Who? Does what? When? With what tools and training?

• Baseline data to be collected?

Ⓔ **DO →What are we learning as we *do* the pilot?**

Ⓕ **CHECK →As we *check* and *study* what happened, what have we learned?**
• Did original outcomes improve?

Ⓖ **ACT →As we *act* to hold the gains or abandon our pilot efforts, what needs to be done?**

Side B of the Clinical Improvement Worksheet invites more focused attention to the development and implementation of specific tests of change in clinical settings.

empowering them to take aim at specific targets in the caregiving process. Attention will be focused on high-leverage areas for tests of change and will occur in a context that supports discussion of care processes and desired outcomes. On the basis of brainstorming work performed in Chapter 2, clinicians might already have a good idea of where improvement efforts should be focused.

1. Outcomes → Select a Population

What is the general aim, and who are we trying to help? Identify a patient population in which there is both strong clinician interest and compelling organizational need. Potential criteria include procedures or diagnoses with high volume, high risk, high cost (including long lengths of stay), high per-case improvement potential, tough market competition, and/or high probability of achieving change. Another important consideration is the perceived relevance of this improvement to patients, clinicians, and other stakeholders.

What are the desired results? State the aim in terms of the specific population selected. What results does the team hope to achieve, and how will they reduce the burden of illness for the target population? Start with a broad statement of the aim, and then focus it on the selected patient population.

Define the Population

On the basis of the general aim statement, brainstorm to identify potentially important clinical, functional, satisfaction, and cost outcomes for the selected patient population. Start with clinical outcomes ("west" on the Clinical Value Compass), proceed to functional health status ("north") and satisfaction against need ("east"), and finish with total costs ("south").

2. Process → Analyze the Process

What is the process for giving care to this type of patient? Construct a flowchart of the care delivery process. Begin by specifying the process boundaries—that is, the steps where this core clinical process starts and finishes for the selected patient population. Specifically define the following:
1. The process starts when patients
_____ (fill in the blank).

2. The process ends when patients
_____ (fill in the blank).

Draft a flowchart of the delivery process by talking through the specific points of action, decision, and transition that characterize a typical patient encounter. Confirm and modify impressions by physically walking through actual steps, as they might be experienced by the patient. Begin with a simple high-level flowchart (5 to 20 steps), and refine it over time.

Specify the patient characteristics that are likely to affect processes of care delivery or that alter the probability of specific patient outcomes. Descriptors that tend to influence processes or outcomes include patient demographics (age, gender, education, language), health parameters (diagnosis, severity of primary diagnosis, comorbidity), and patient preferences (treatment expectations, lifestyle choices, and valuation of specific results).

3. Changes → Generate Change Ideas

What ideas do we have for changing what is done (the process) to get better results? Think about the aim, the desired results (clinical, functional, satisfaction, costs), and the delivery process (as represented in a flowchart). Targeting problems that have been identified, brainstorm as many changes as possible that could improve care or lower costs. Search the literature to learn from the successes and failures of other similar improvement efforts. Discuss what similar institutions have done. Clarify the ideas generated and determine the most promising change idea for pilot testing.

4. Pilot → Select a Change for Pilot Testing

How can we pilot test an improvement idea? Because not all changes lead to improvement, innovations must be tested to ensure that they add value to the core clinical process. Ask whether, and how, participants can pilot test one idea using the PDSA (Plan–Do–Study–Act) method. If possible, the best tests of change are performed quickly and on a small scale. Now is the time to identify logistical, political, or timing issues that might support or hinder implementation of the pilot test.

Aim . . . Fire . . . Hit (or Miss)

Side B of the Clinical Improvement Worksheet (Figure 3-1, page 25) focuses further attention on a specific test of change. The left side of the worksheet invites participants to reflect on the composition of their team and on specific aims, measures, and characteristics of the selected change. Individually, and in conference with team members, consider the following questions:

1. *Team Members:* Who should work on this improvement?
2. Step A, *Specific Aim:* What are we trying to accomplish?
3. Step B, *Measures:* How will we know whether a change is an improvement?
4. Step C, *Selected Change:* How would we describe the change that we have selected for testing?

Team Members → Who Should Work on This Improvement?

From the original group identified, or among other individuals not previously considered, who needs to be directly involved in this work, and who does not? Use the improvement worksheet to refine thinking about who is needed on the team. Identify team members and choose an appropriate leader. Participants might also wish to name a facilitator, a recordkeeper, and a timekeeper, whose roles can rotate from meeting to meeting. Ancillary team resources should be identified as well, including administrators and coaches, who coordinate or serve as improvement resources across several teams and improvement efforts. Sidebar 3-2, below, presents further discussion of team formation and effective team meetings. Chapter 8 expands on teamwork and collaboration.

Specific Aim → What Are We Trying to Accomplish?

What specifically is the team trying to accomplish with this test of change? Make a more definite and structured aim statement that clarifies intentions, expectations, and priorities. This aim will guide subsequent planning and self-assessment of the proposed pilot study.

To help sharpen the aim statement, complete the following sentences:

1. The aim is to improve the quality and value of _____ (name of clinical care process).

Sidebar 3-2. Improvement Team Meeting Process and Holding Effective Meetings

Because time is a precious resource for practitioners of clinical improvement, efficient and effective team meetings will optimize the active and intelligent participation of all team members. Leaders of such groups might wish to educate themselves in the principles and methods of team formation, team function, and productive and enjoyable team meetings. Much has been written on this topic. *The Team Handbook,* by Scholtes, Joiner, and Streibel, is an excellent resource.[*] Another helpful resource is Chapter 12, "Effective Meeting Skills 1" in the textbook *Quality by Design: A Clinical Microsystems Approach* by Nelson, Batalden, and Godfrey.[†] Some key points follow:

1. Plan to meet regularly and have a regular schedule (day, time, and place to meet) so that meeting becomes a part of the team members' routine.
2. Identify common meeting roles to help team members become more aware of their work and more skilled in meeting tasks. It is helpful to rotate the meeting roles so that each team member can gain insight into the importance of each role and practice the skills.
3. The four essential meeting roles are leader, timekeeper, recorder, and facilitator. These roles can be combined, but keeping roles separated when a group first begins to hold meetings helps everyone understand the benefits of a group process.
4. A meeting is a process of three steps: (1) the premeeting phase, in which the date, time, and agenda are set; (2) the in-meeting, in which the team focuses and works on objectives; and (3) the postmeeting phase, in which members follow through on decisions and create an agenda for the next meeting.
5. Meetings should have preset ground rules discussed and agreed on by all team members. It is helpful to periodically assess how well meetings are following the ground rules.

References

[*] Scholtes PR, Joiner BL, Streibel BJ. *The Team Handbook,* 3rd ed. Madison, WI: Oriel, 2003.
[†] Nelson EC, Batalden PB, Godfrey MM, editors. *Quality by Design: A Clinical Microsystems Approach.* San Francisco: Jossey-Bass, 2007.

2. This clinical care process starts with _____ _____ (starting point of the process), and the process ends when _____ (end point of the process).

3. By working on this process, we expect to improve _____ (the anticipated better outcomes).

4. It is important to work on this process now because _____(reasons that make this process important from the perspective of the patient, clinician, or purchaser of care).

Measures → How Will We Know Whether a Change Is an Improvement?

A few balanced measures can be used to evaluate the success (outcomes and costs) and potential adverse effects or unintended consequences of the pilot. Measures should flow from the specific aim statement cited in Step A on Side B of the worksheet and from the more general, higher-level list of outcomes generated in Step 1 on Side A.

Selected Change → How Would We Describe the Change That We Have Selected for Testing?

Describe the change that has been selected for testing, and use this spot on the improvement worksheet to keep track of other potential changes the team might wish to try in the future. The essence of continual improvement is to run repeated, rapid, and increasingly effective tests of change.

PDSA Cycle

The right column of Side B of the Clinical Improvement Worksheet (Figure 3-1, page 25) outlines the basic steps of a PDSA improvement cycle as the second half of the series of improvement steps begun in the left column. Having taken aim at a specific improvement target, team members are empowered in the PDSA cycle to fire more accurately and to determine whether each shot was a hit or a miss. The cycle challenges participants to address (through action) the following essential questions:

1. Step D, *Plan:* How shall we plan the pilot?
2. Step E, *Do:* What are we learning as we do the pilot?
3. Step F, *Study:* As we study what happened, what have we learned?
4. Step G, *Act:* As we act to hold the gains or abandon our pilot efforts, what needs to be done?

Plan → How Shall We Plan the Pilot?

What is the plan and how will it be implemented? In essence, define who does what and when. Also define the tools and training needed to implement the pilot (if any). Write a brief change protocol that answers these questions and then illustrate the protocol with a simple flowchart. A good plan must be executed well to succeed; participants involved should know what they are doing and why they are doing it. Flowchart illustrations can be beneficial here.

Baseline data should be collected. Write a brief data collection protocol indicating who will gather and analyze what data from what sources. Use precise operational definitions so that all participants speak the same language and enact the same protocol.

Do → What Are We Learning as We Do the Pilot?

Keep a diary of the pilot project, open to reflections from all participants. Comment on whether discrete steps and the intervention as a whole are proceeding as planned. The results of this pilot will be no better than the care with which the planned change was executed. Observations about the process can help prepare the way for making more powerful changes in the future.

Study → As We Study What Happened, What Have We Learned?

Did original outcomes improve? Were any unintended consequences or adverse outcomes observed? Analyze the pilot test results in a way that answers the main question: Did the change lead to the predicted improvement?

Act → As We Act to Hold the Gains or Abandon Our Pilot Efforts, What Needs to Be Done?

If the pilot was successful, the next task is to incorporate this positive change into daily work routines, so that ongoing delivery of care proceeds efficiently and effectively. If the pilot was not successful, then analyze the source(s) of this failure and welcome this new opportunity to learn. Failure is an invitation to generate new theories of cause and effect. Do not be discouraged. Many tests of change will fail to produce the desired positive result, but all such tests can stimulate insight that supports future, and perhaps more effective, clinical improvement.

Using the Clinical Improvement Worksheet: Improving the Care of Adolescent Kidney Transplant Recipients

A renal transplant physician at a large academic hospital in Toronto noted the high rates of patient nonadherence and poor outcomes in adolescent kidney transplant recipients. The story of a real patient, Amber, described in Sidebar 3-1 (page 22) illustrated the concept. The physician believed that the existing transfer process between pediatric and adult care was poorly coordinated and was contributing to these poor results. Figure 3-2 (page 30) shows a completed Side A of the Renal Transplant Transition Clinical Improvement Worksheet, highlighting the team's efforts. The description that follows illustrates the process of how a renal transplant team developed an innovative idea to improve care during this transition period.

Team Members → Who Should Work on This Improvement?

The Renal Transplant Transition Team that was formed consists of an adult nephrologist, a pediatric nephrologist, an adolescent medicine specialist, a transplant coordinator at each hospital site, and a pediatric nurse practitioner. Although a patient was not initially involved as a team member, team members learned that patient input was a crucial component for identifying barriers faced.

Outcomes → Select a Population

Nonadherence with immunosuppressive medications is common, occurring in a quarter of kidney transplant recipients, and is associated with poor outcomes. Adolescents are at particularly high risk for nonadherence. While short-term graft survival in adolescents is excellent, five-year graft survival rates are poorer than in any other age group except those older than 65 years of age.[4] The period of transition between pediatric and adult care has been identified as a high-risk period for nonadherence among adolescent kidney transplant recipients. Inadequate immunosuppression causes graft failure and requires treatment for rejection. Return to dialysis is associated with a decrease in quality of life and increased health care utilization and costs. Thus, the clinical team had identified a patient population with a well-defined need, for whom intervention was likely to yield meaningful improvement.

The goal of the transition team was to improve outcomes and to reduce costs for adolescent renal transplant recipients. The outcomes for each of the four Clinical Value Compass points are the following:

- **Clinical Outcomes:** graft survival, renal failure
- **Functional Health Status:** nonadherence behavior, daily ability to go to work or school, mood, ability to participate in extracurricular activities
- **Satisfaction Against Need:** perceived health status, satisfaction with transfer process
- **Total Costs:** missed clinic appointments, emergency department use and hospital admissions, rejection treatment, dialysis, lost tuition fees, and lost productivity for the patient and family members

A Renal Transplant Transition Clinical Value Compass annotated with selected measures was created (Figure 3-3, page 31).

Process → Analyze the Process

Prior to the initiation of the transition clinic, it was the responsibility of the individual pediatric nephrologist to refer each patient to one of six adult transplant nephrologists at his or her 18th birthday. Information was communicated to the accepting

Figure 3-2. Completed Clinical Improvement Worksheet: Renal Transplant Transition

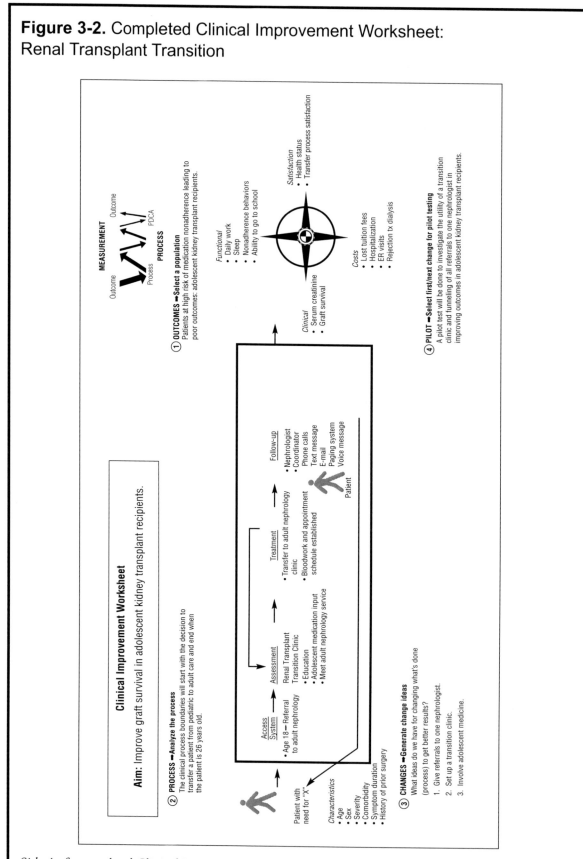

Side A of a completed Clinical Improvement Worksheet illustrates progress made by the Renal Transplant Transition Team.

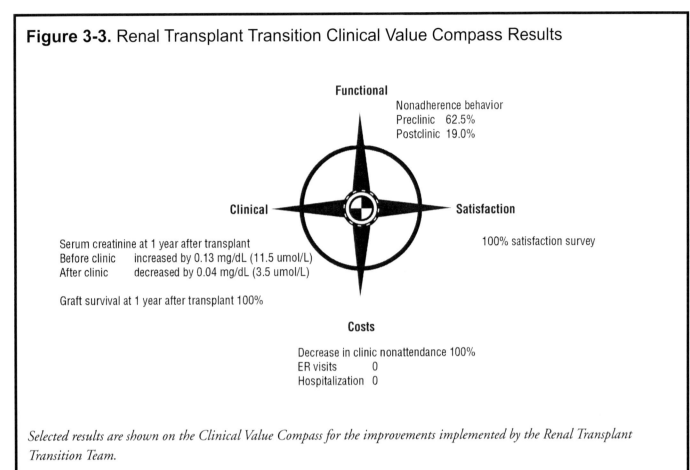

Figure 3-3. Renal Transplant Transition Clinical Value Compass Results

Functional

Nonadherence behavior
Preclinic   62.5%
Postclinic 19.0%

Clinical

Satisfaction

100% satisfaction survey

Serum creatinine at 1 year after transplant
Before clinic   increased by 0.13 mg/dL (11.5 umol/L)
After clinic   decreased by 0.04 mg/dL (3.5 umol/L)

Graft survival at 1 year after transplant 100%

Costs

Decrease in clinic nonattendance 100%
ER visits   0
Hospitalization 0

Selected results are shown on the Clinical Value Compass for the improvements implemented by the Renal Transplant Transition Team.

Reproduced with permission from The Dartmouth Institute for Health Policy and Clinical Practice (TDI).

physician in a transfer letter. There was no formal orientation to the adult care setting for adolescent patients and their families, nor did patients meet with their new adult care providers prior to transfer. The transfer process therefore began with the last appointment at the pediatric hospital and ended with the first appointment in the adult care setting. The team developed and charted a process map.

Changes → Generate Change Ideas

During the improvement process, the team generated and discussed many ideas. The Renal Transplant Transition Clinic was implemented as a joint initiative between the pediatric and adult care providers. The transition process begins two years before transfer. The clinic provides a structured meeting between the patient and the new adult care team, consisting of a transplant nephrologist and a nurse specialist transplant coordinator. Patients and parents separately participate in small-group discussions facilitated by adolescent

medicine team members, meet their new adult providers, complete a health summary, and receive an information booklet on transferring to adult care and a graduation certificate. All referrals are directed to a single adult transplant nephrologist, who attends the transition clinic and is responsible for all adolescent patients upon transfer. Patients continue to attend the transition clinic until the age of 24 years, as this is the time period in which they are considered to be at high risk for nonadherence and graft rejection.

Pilot → Select a Change for Pilot Testing

The two main changes piloted were the following:

1. Transition clinic initiated prior to transfer of care
2. All referrals directed to one adult transplant nephrologist

It was hypothesized that this change would result in improved medication adherence, greater patient satisfaction, reductions in health costs, and better clinical outcomes.

Specific Aim → What Are We Trying to Accomplish?

The aim of the Renal Transplant Transition Team was to improve graft survival in adolescent kidney transplant recipients.

Measures → How Will We Know Whether a Change Is an Improvement?

The team decided to focus on two clinical outcomes (serum creatinine, graft survival), one functional outcome (nonadherence), and satisfaction. Direct costs were not initially included. Given that a well-accepted definition for *nonadherence* was available for patients with renal transplant, the team decided to develop a specific definition (that is, an operational definition). The team defined *nonadherence* as either self-reported medication nonadherence or displaying at least two of the following three characteristics: nonattendance at clinic, nonattendance for blood-work appointments, or undetectable measures of cyclosporin, a medication to prevent rejection.

Clinical outcomes were examined by measuring change in serum creatinine at one year after transfer to the adult clinic and monitoring the incidence of rejection. Patient satisfaction prior to and after the intervention was assessed by a self-administered questionnaire. Later on during the process and as a proxy for measuring health care costs, we explored nonattendance at clinic, emergency department visits, and hospital admissions.

Selected Change → How Would We Describe the Change That We Have Selected for Testing?

The initiative included the aforementioned transition clinic and follow-up of all adolescent patients by a single transplant nephrologist following transfer to adult care. The choice for the selected change was based on other successful transition clinics described in the literature.

To measure the effect of this change, baseline data were extracted from the pediatric renal transplant database, and parameters of graft function and adherence were measured in a prospective fashion following transfer.

Plan → How Shall We Plan the Pilot?

The team decided on the following steps necessary for the pilot study:

- Dates and location for the transition clinic agreed upon
- Budgetary implications of intervention determined
- Staff educated
- Health care participants identified
- Patients selected
- Data collected and compiled
- Measures identified

Do → What Are We Learning as We Do the Pilot?

During the pilot intervention, the Renal Transplant Transition Team members discovered that preclinic planning and coordination were key to the success of the initiative. This multidisciplinary clinic required the expertise of several specialties and disciplines, and it was thus impractical for the clinic to occur more than twice yearly. This scheduling raised logistic issues in dealing with patient cancellations. The involvement of an adolescent medicine specialist led to higher-than-anticipated rates of patient disclosure of self-reported medication nonadherence, affecting its validity as an outcome measure. In addition, it highlighted the need for continued involvement of an adolescent medicine specialist after transfer.

Study → As We Study What Happened, What Have We Learned?

To determine the impact of change, the team analyzed the first 16 patients who transferred to the adult care setting after implementation of the initiative. Specific outcomes were as follows:

- **Clinical:** The mean serum creatinine of patients who had attended the transition clinic fell by 0.04 mg/dL (or 3.5 umol/L) in the first year. In comparison, the mean serum creatinine of the last 16 patients to transfer prior to initiation of the clinic had increased by 0.13 mg/dL (11.5 umol/L). Graft survival at 12 months was

100%. As no longitudinal follow-up existed before the implementation of this clinic, graft survival had not been previously tracked.

- **Functional:** The incidence of nonadherent behavior was 19% in the group transferring after the described changes were made—a decrease from a nonadherence rate of 62.5% prior to the work of the Renal Transplant Transition Team.
- **Satisfaction:** Patient satisfaction was 100%.
- **Costs:** The exact cost was not calculated; however, there were only 4 missed appointments in the first year, compared to 18 in the previous year. There were no emergency department visits.

Act → As We Act to Hold the Gains or Abandon Our Pilot Efforts, What Needs to Be Done?

The team and hospital administration concluded that the pilot test was successful. The further plan for the transition clinic is to expand the number of patients it cares for in the area. Other opportunities not described here further arose, such as the transition of care of children with chronic kidney disease who were not yet on renal replacement therapy.

Moving Forward

The Clinical Improvement Worksheet has been used in ambulatory and hospital settings, in intensive care units,[5] and as part of training program curricula[6] to address improvement in primary prevention, acute surgical care, and posthospital rehabilitation. The instrument is useful whenever a specific clinical population can be identified that undergoes a more or less predictable clinical process. On the basis of our and others' experience with the improvement worksheet, we offer the following strategies for optimal implementation:

- *Think of ramping up improvements.* Improvement teams will benefit from conceptualizing their short-term work in longer-term contexts. Think about running repeated tests of change over time rather than finding the quick fix. Figure 3-4 (page 34)

depicts a continual improvement ramp in which small, rapid tests of change support one another sequentially. A first test of change might be to standardize a single small step in a larger process that varies significantly. In the example of the Renal Transplant Transition Clinic, this could be the change in referral pattern of adolescent patients from multiple physicians to a single nephrologist. This might be followed by a second change in which the order of steps is modified so that delays are prevented downstream. A third change might be more substantial, such as the development of standing orders or care guidelines to clarify more generally the interventions that must occur during each stage of the process flow.

- *Conduct each test to unsettle the existing system and to provide useful information on the design of further change.* With time, as more and more trials are conducted, the complexity of interventions might increase as experience with successful change accumulates. In the example of the Renal Transplant Transition Clinic, an initial improvement was to establish a database to collate and review blood results from different laboratories attended by geographically disparate patients. A team might progress from simple, small improvements (with real but modest impact on quality and value) to total process redesign and radical reengineering (with a very large impact on quality and value). Participants often arrive at their first meeting with many ideas for improvement—these are usually the obvious changes. As the team ascends its ramp of sequential improvements, the breadth and depth of potential interventions expands in concert with increasing process knowledge itself.

- *Accelerate tests of change.* Although improvement work takes practice, the aim should be rapid redesign. With experience, both the number and the speed of change cycles can increase. Cutting *cycle time* (that is, time from conceptualization of the change concept to conclusion of a small-scale pilot test) should be a practice objective. Indeed, this cycle time can itself be the object of measurement, motivating teams to improve their very process of improvement. Setting an ambitious timetable early in the work can help pick up the pace of change.

- *Think of multiple ways to make improvements.* The Clinical Improvement Worksheet is versatile. Its foundational question—"What ideas do we have for changing what is done to get better results?"—invites people to think broadly about change concepts that might produce better outcomes. A *change concept* is a general notion or approach to change that is useful in developing specific ideas for clinical improvement.[7] For example, if the change concept is "standardization," ideas for change might include development of clinical guidelines or design of a critical pathway. Change concepts are discussed further in Chapter 6.

Implementation in the Real World

Implementing changes can be challenging. Most of us suffer from "change-process illiteracy." We have only limited knowledge of how things really work in our own practices, and what we do know is not documented. This lack of knowledge of "what is" impedes our ability to design "what should be." To make matters worse, we often fail to understand and anticipate resistance to change among colleagues who must be involved (at the front line and in the front office) if clinical innovations are to be successful.

Thus, to facilitate positive change in clinical practice, improvement teams must maximize their understanding of current care processes, and leaders of improvement work must be skilled in managing the interpersonal dimensions of process change. Chapter 8 expands on concepts to build teamwork and enhance collaboration. Chapter 9 provides a broader perspective of implementing change.

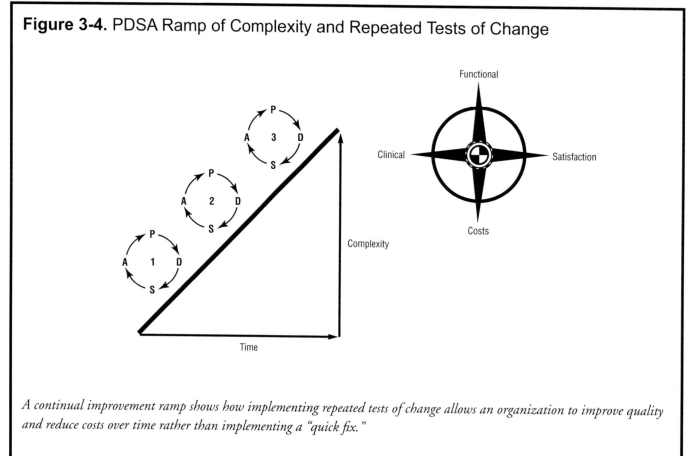

Figure 3-4. PDSA Ramp of Complexity and Repeated Tests of Change

A continual improvement ramp shows how implementing repeated tests of change allows an organization to improve quality and reduce costs over time rather than implementing a "quick fix."

PDSA: Plan–Do–Study–Act.

Visualizing the Core Clinical Process

Improvement teams find great value in diagramming the core clinical process and then in addressing each component of this process in turn. In general, activities proceed sequentially in all or most clinical settings: access, assessment, diagnosis, treatment, and follow-up. Improvement in performance can be achieved by understanding the core clinical process and systematically identifying sources of variability, delays, or waste that occur at various stages.[8] Thus, for example, an ambulatory care visit for severe sore throat might be diagrammed as a core clinical process that includes the following discrete steps: patient calls practice for an appointment; appointment is scheduled; patient checks in with receptionist; medical assistant takes patient to examination room and obtains chief complaint and vital signs; clinician obtains history, performs targeted examination, and orders a confirmatory laboratory test; patient receives education on home care and treatment plan; patient adheres (or does not adhere) to treatment plan; and practice contacts patient (or vice versa) three days after visit to assess progress and to plan follow-up care.

This parsing of even a "straightforward" core clinical process will often reveal multiple targets for improvement. We advise teams to analyze and to map their own clinical activities in these terms and then to attach performance measures to each identified component of the core process. Data can be gathered on key upstream measures to determine their specific relationship to measures farther downstream.

In addition, teams can use deployment flowcharts to plan and to monitor the implementation process itself.[9] Even simple tests of change often require substantial coordination. In the example of the Renal Transplant Transition Clinic, ensuring that all adolescent patients be seen in future visits by one nephrologist resulted in unforeseen logistical requirements, including the necessity for a dedicated transition coordinator for transplant recipients. Deployment flowcharts identify specific actors and actions at each step in the redesigned clinical process. Constructing this flowchart facilitates communication between all participants and optimizes sequential handoffs (of both information and patient care responsibility) from one team member to the next.

Managing Change

All clinical change occurs in an interpersonal context and is supported or impeded by both the individual motivations and the collective dynamics of the organization. Even the best-conceived improvement plans will falter if the motivations and dynamics are not effectively managed. We have used and modified several change management guidelines on the basis of the work of Kotter,[10] Reinertsen,[11] and others. The following guidelines are illustrated in reference to the Renal Transplant Transition Clinic:

1. *Understand and communicate the cost of the status quo.* The transition team compared current nonadherence, missed appointments, and graft failure with the expected new outcomes, data that motivated participants to embrace the new way.

2. *Develop and communicate the specific vision of a better way.* The transition team articulated and operationalized its vision in the course of sequential meetings and involved stakeholders from all areas, including transplant nephrologists, nurse coordinators, and adolescent medicine specialists, ensuring collective ownership of the new intervention.

3. *Obtain the commitment of those with the power to make the new way legitimate.* The adult transplant nephrologists agreed that centralizing care ensured an improved transition process.

4. *Make sure that the change agents have the skills to achieve both human and technical objectives and ensure that individuals are supported and recognized for their work.* Transition team members supported and recognized one another, and they worked with each patient to ensure comfort with the transition to adult care.

5. *Anticipate, understand, and manage the resistance to achieve commitment.* The transition team involved physicians specialized in adolescent medicine to identify key barriers to completing transition.

6. *Align change with the organization's culture.* The organization is working to emphasize high-value clinical care, and the new transition team's aim was therefore well aligned with this goal.

7. *Leave enough organizational "change reserve" to handle unexpected events.* The transition team focused on first testing the concept on a small scale before proceeding to implementation.

8. *Prepare a thorough change management plan.* The transition team developed a flowchart and time line to clarify all essential steps in the anticipated test of change.

Linking Improvement Work to Meaningful Clinical Outcomes

The Clinical Improvement Worksheet supports development of tests of change in diverse practice settings. In this chapter we have traveled with one clinical team as it implemented and learned from a specific improvement initiative. Patient-oriented outcomes are the driving force for all such initiatives, defining particular targets for improvement and specifying performance measures for ongoing assessment. The Clinical Improvement Worksheet can also be used as a guide and template to organize and communicate improvement efforts in clinical medicine[12–14] and in scientific publications.[5,15–18] Also, the worksheet can assist in education for health professionals, including residents in training and interprofessional education. [19–21]

Chapter 4 expands the description and utility of the Clinical Value Compass, a tool that complements the Clinical Improvement Worksheet, to monitor outcomes that are most meaningful to patients (and their families), health care practitioners, and systems.

References

1. McInnis D. What system? *Dartmouth Medicine.* 2006;30(4):28–35.

2. Nelson EC, et al.: Improving health care, Part 1: The Clinical Value Compass. *Jt Comm J Qual Improv.* 1996 Apr;22(4):243–258.

3. Versteeg MH, et al. Factors associated with the impact of quality improvement collaboratives in mental healthcare: An exploratory study. *Implement Sci.* 2012 Jan 9;7:1.

4. Magee JC, et al. Pediatric transplantation. *Am J Transplant.* 2004;4 Suppl 9:54–57.

5. Wall RJ, et al. Using real time process measurements to reduce catheter related bloodstream infections in the intensive care unit. *Qual Saf Health Care.* 2005 Aug;14(4):295–302.

6. Mohr JJ, et al. Integrating improvement competencies into residency education: A pilot project from a pediatric continuity clinic. *Ambul Pediatr.* 2003 May–Jun;3(3):131–136.

7. Langley GJ, et al. *The Improvement Guide: A Practical Approach to Enhancing Organizational Performance,* 2nd ed. San Francisco: Jossey-Bass, 2009.

8. Chand S, et al. Improving patient flow at an outpatient clinic: Study of sources of variability and improvement factors. *Health Care Manag Sci.* 2009 Sep;12(3):325–340.

9. Scholtes PR, Joiner BL, Streibel BJ. *The Team Handbook,* 3rd ed. Madison, WI: Oriel, 2003.

10. Kotter JP. *Leading Change.* Boston: Harvard Business School Press, 1996.

11. Reinertsen J. Improving clinical quality. Paper presented at the American Group Practice Association Annual Meeting, New Orleans, 1995.

12. Plsek PE. Quality improvement methods in clinical medicine. *Pediatrics.* 1999 Jan;103(1 Suppl E):203–214.

13. Focht A, Jones AE, Lowe TJ. Early goal-directed therapy: Improving mortality and morbidity of sepsis in the emergency department. *Jt Comm J Qual Patient Saf.* 2009 Apr;35(4):186–191.

14. Puskarich MA, et al. One year mortality of patients treated with an emergency department based early goal directed therapy protocol for severe sepsis and septic shock: A before and after study. *Crit Care.* 2009;13(5):R167.

15. Ogrinc G, et al. The SQUIRE (Standards for QUality Improvement Reporting Excellence) guidelines for quality improvement reporting: Explanation and elaboration. *Qual Saf Health Care.* 2008 Oct;17 Suppl 1:i13–32.

16. White DE, et al. What is the value and impact of quality and safety teams? A scoping review. *Implement Sci.* 2011 Aug 23;6:97.

17. Chaboyer W, et al. Redesigning the ICU nursing discharge process: A quality improvement study. *Worldviews Evid Based Nurs.* 2012 Feb;9(1):40–48.

18. Horbar JD, et al. Collaborative quality improvement to promote evidence based surfactant for preterm infants: A cluster randomised trial. *BMJ.* 2004 Oct 30;329(7473):1004.

19. Cooke M, Ironside PM, Ogrinc GS. Mainstreaming quality and safety: A reformulation of quality and safety education for health professions students. *BMJ Qual Saf.* 2011 Apr;20 Suppl 1:i79–i82.

20. Oujiri J, et al. Resident-initiated interventions to improve inpatient heart-failure management. *BMJ Qual Saf.* 2011 Feb;20(2):181–186.

21. Wilcock PM, Campion-Smith C, Head M. The Dorset Seedcorn Project: Interprofessional learning and continuous quality improvement in primary care. *Br J Gen Pract.* 2002 Oct;52 Suppl:S39–S44.

Chapter 4

MEASURING OUTCOMES AND COSTS: THE CLINICAL VALUE COMPASS

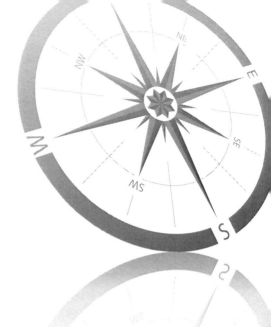

Mark E. Splaine, Anne C. Jones, Eugene C. Nelson, Julie K. Johnson, Paul B. Batalden

When you can measure what you are speaking about, and express it in numbers, you know something about it; but when you cannot measure it, when you cannot express it in numbers, your knowledge is of a meagre and unsatisfactory kind; it may be the beginning of knowledge, but you have scarcely in your thoughts advanced to the stage of Science.

—Lord Kelvin[1]

Health care providers are getting a wake-up call. Outcome-based measures of clinical performance (for hospitals, ambulatory care organizations, and even individual practitioners) are increasingly transparent to public scrutiny, and the payment structure for clinical services continues a rapid shift toward "value-based" purchasing. The concept of value itself, once an abstraction, has been operationalized by private insurers, commercial employers, and now Medicare as well, in "pay-for-performance" models of reimbursement.[2] Both patients and purchasers seek high-quality care at low cost and increasingly align themselves with health care providers and health systems that can meet this demand. Clinicians in this new century will need to demonstrate value and to continually improve it to realize full payment for services rendered.

Real improvement and real value in health care depend on a linking of patient priorities and system processes to specific outcome measurements. The Clinical Value Compass, introduced in earlier chapters, provides a conceptual framework that precisely links values of patients and clinicians to the measurable value that health care systems provide. In this chapter we further develop the notion of health care value, and we explore the utility of the Clinical Value Compass

for understanding and monitoring clinical processes and outcomes in a variety of patient care settings. Our aim is to stimulate readers' use and adaptation of this model in their own work.

Health Care Value

The concept of health care value has continued to gain increasing acceptance among patients, practitioners, and other stakeholders in the delivery of clinical services. The motto might be put simply: "Best quality. Lowest cost. No excuses!"[3] The era of value in health care is now upon us, with *value* defined as a relationship between quality received (or provided) and costs incurred in the receipt (or provision) of that quality.[4] This relationship can be formalized in a simple equation:

$$\text{Value} = f\ (\text{Quality} \div \text{Costs})$$

In other words, the value of a clinical service is directly proportional to the quality of that service (or the quality of benefits that arise from that service) and inversely proportional to the costs associated with that same service. Thus, as costs of an intervention go up, the value goes down, even when quality is held constant.

The advantage of this simple formula is that its basic terms are relevant to, and appropriately understood by, all stakeholders in health care relationships, from patients and clinicians to employers and insurers. From the perspective of health care providers and purchasers, the total cost to the system can be conceptualized more precisely as the product of unit costs and volume, as in the following more detailed equation:

Total costs to system = (costs per unit volume) × (volume of unit services provided or received)

Thus, in a technical sense, both these terms (unit costs and volume) appear in the denominator of the value equation. From the patient's perspective, however, volume is almost always "1" (that is, the patient himself or herself), in which case the more detailed equation reduces to the simpler and more intuitive version offered first.

Those who pay for health care, particularly employers and insurers (but also individual patients, who bear a growing proportion of this burden), focus increasingly on value defined in precisely these terms. The concept of *value-based purchasing* is now widely used and understood. Those who provide clinical service, from individual practitioners to regional hospital networks, recognize the imperative to concentrate similarly on value-based care. This imperative is rooted in the ethical principle that professionals should improve their work and the financial principle that the ongoing escalation of health care costs needs to be addressed.

There is skepticism in some quarters about whether quality and value can be accurately quantified in real-world clinical settings. Great advances have been made, however, in the measurement of health status, health risk, and patient satisfaction.[5] We believe that measuring quality and outcomes is no longer an insurmountable barrier in the documentation of clinical improvement. On the contrary, such measurement is not only practicable but also essential in continuous improvement work.

Wise application of continual improvement methods can generate better value in health care settings, just as it has enhanced quality and reduced costs in other sectors of the economy.[6] The Clinical Value Compass integrates components of quality and value that all stakeholders can recognize as important, and it thus empowers the health care team to develop and sustain meaningful improvements in a wide variety of patient care contexts.

The Clinical Value Compass Approach

We base our discussion of health care value on a series of assumptions that are shared by most patients, clinicians, and payers of health services. These assumptions include the following general principles:

- The aim of health care is to maintain health and wellness as well as to prevent, to diagnose, and to treat disease, and thereby to reduce or limit the burden of illness through restoration, maintenance, or improvement of health functioning.[7–9]
- Health is experienced simultaneously in biologic, psychological, functional, and social dimensions.[10]
- Quality health care provides the services (that is, clinical care processes) that are most likely to achieve desired health outcomes at a price that represents value for the patient.[4]
- The value of health care is a function of both quality and costs (per unit volume of service provided or received).[4,11]

How can we pull these assumptions together into a useful, understandable whole? Many models have been applied, but we find particular utility in the value compass approach. As introduced in Chapters 1 and 3 and depicted again in Figure 4-1 (page 39), the value compass approach honors multiple components of patient-defined value and recognizes shifts in these values over time. At the conceptual center of the value compass are individuals or populations who, at a specific point in time, experience a new or continuing health care need (for example, a middle-aged man requires acute management of myocardial infarction, an elderly woman seeks treatment for recurrent depression, or parents desire routine immunization for their young child as part of routine preventive care). These patients can be described as being at *baseline*—before a treatment episode begins—in terms of their clinical (biologic) status, functional health and risk status, and expectations (what they hope health care can accomplish for them in terms of pain relief, symptom reduction, freedom from physical and mental limitations, and so forth). The patients can also be characterized by the health-related costs incurred over time for management of each particular need. These costs include both direct expenses for medical care and indirect social expenses (including time lost from work) that arise from management of the illness burden or preventive care. In an important sense, the cost meter for each individual starts running at birth and continues rising until death, taking a jump with each episode of new health need.

The Clinical Value Compass in Figure 4-1 also illustrates the flow of the health care delivery process: the patient accessing the system, then caregivers assessing, diagnosing, treating, and following up with the patient in need. These process steps create a result for each patient or population that can be measured in terms of specific quality-related outcomes and costs. As described in Chapter 3, these outcomes are in fact transitions in quality-related health status (clinical condition, function, satisfaction) and incremental costs associated with treatment over time.

We call the circular display of measures—depicted twice in Figure 4-1 (pre-episode and postepisode)—the Clinical Value Compass because the layout resembles an old-fashioned, directional compass used for navigation. It has four cardinal points:

- **West:** clinical or biologic outcomes (for example, mortality, morbidity, complications)
- **North:** functional health status, risk status, and well-being
- **East:** expectation of health outcomes (pre-episode) and satisfaction with health care and perceived health benefit (postepisode)
- **South:** costs, both direct (for example, health care costs for physicians, hospitals, drugs) and indirect (for example, social costs incurred by the family, employer, community)

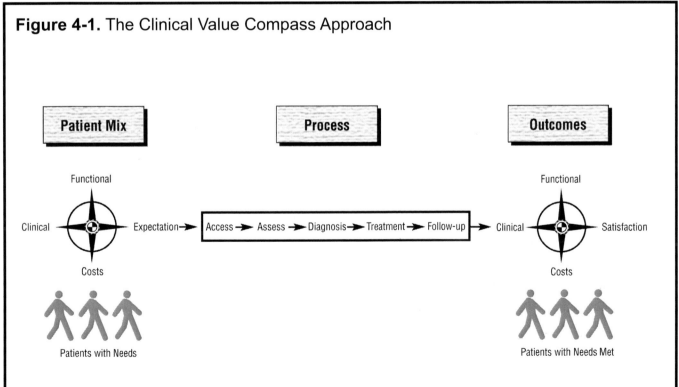

Figure 4-1. The Clinical Value Compass Approach

The Clinical Value Compass illustrates the flow of the care-delivery process and its results.

This heuristic model barely begins to capture the rich complexity of patient experiences and clinical services in real-world settings. A truly comprehensive assessment of quality and value would map multiple dimensions of health system structure (facilities, equipment, supplies, personnel) and process (safety, appropriateness, availability, continuity, effectiveness, efficacy, respect, timeliness) against various outcomes of clinical relevance (biologic function, mental health, social/occupational capacity, health risk status, health-related quality of life) and would extend this mapping to all particular health concerns that might arise in a patient's life (low back pain, depression, chemical dependency, pregnancy and childbirth, and so on). But such an assessment would be costly and prohibitively complex. The Clinical Value Compass simplifies this process, inviting practitioners to select critical indicators of process and outcome known to be important to specific patient populations and to focus attention on improvement in these domains over time.

Finally, we wish to emphasize that we use the value compass as a metaphor to bring to mind four aspects of health care value—clinical status, functional health and risk status, satisfaction, and costs—just as a compass brings to mind the four cardinal points of west, north, east, and south. Like the physical compass used for ocean navigation or for backcountry orienteering, the conceptual compass of clinical value specifies no inherent hierarchy of its points. All are important. The landscape in all directions is open to exploration, appreciation, and improvement.

But no metaphor is perfect, and some individuals might find the compass image confusing. Directional arrows seem to "pull" in opposite directions and suggest to some users that gains in one territory must be achieved through loss in the several others. Certainly, clinicians are familiar with perceived tensions between high-quality patient care and the economic bottom line or between patient satisfaction and the rigorous demands of disease management. If we consider the interests of other stakeholders, including employers and other health care purchasers, the potential for conflict might be even greater.

Our own experience, however, is that these very tensions can generate creative solutions beneficial to all stakeholders. The Clinical Value Compass appeals not only to patients and their practitioners but also to employers and stakeholders precisely because it invites a balancing of perspectives and priorities. Cooperation rather than conflict can flourish if all parties gain a deeper appreciation of their common interest in high-value care. Most stakeholders want patients to enjoy an active, productive, independent life, and most want to ensure that appropriate clinical care occurs in a satisfying and efficient manner. In addition, controlling unnecessary costs—including health care costs that do not add value—meets the needs of providers, patients, employers, and purchasers.

Our patients, in the end, do not experience themselves as travelers in discrete quadrants of biologic, functional, psychological, and financial reality. They live instead as integrated persons at the junction of these several domains. The circle that draws together these distinct elements of the Clinical Value Compass reminds us, as clinical experience confirms, that creative work in one domain almost always connects to and stimulates improvement in several others. Real value in health care is achievable in terms that are common to all stakeholders.

Clinical Value Compass Worksheet

As discussed in greater detail in Chapter 3, practitioners who wish to manage and to improve the value of their clinical services will benefit from participation in the following cycle of reflective work:

- Measuring the value of care in specific patient populations
- Analyzing the internal delivery processes that contribute significantly to current levels of measured outcomes and costs
- Running tests of change in delivery processes
- Determining whether these changes lead to better outcomes and lower costs

The worksheet presented in Figure 4-2 (page 41) aids clinicians in this improvement process. The worksheet helps individuals efficiently identify key

Figure 4-2. Clinical Value Compass Worksheet, Side A

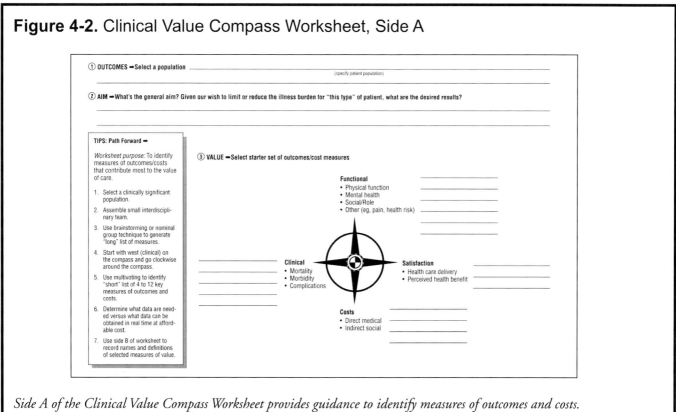

Side A of the Clinical Value Compass Worksheet provides guidance to identify measures of outcomes and costs.

Source: Reproduced with permission from The Dartmouth Institute for Health Policy and Clinical Practice (TDI).

Figure 4-2. Clinical Value Compass Worksheet, Side B

④ SPECIFIC OPERATIONAL DEFINITIONS ➡ for key outcome and cost measures

TIPS: Writing Definitions ➡

A *conceptual definition* is a brief statement describing a variable of interest. It should tell people <u>what</u> you want to measure and who "owns" it.

An *operational definition* is a clearly specified <u>method</u> for reliably sorting, classifying, or measuring a variable. It should be written as an instruction set, or protocol, that would enable two different people to measure the variable by using the same process and thereby producing the same result. It should explain to people <u>how</u> a variable should be measured.

Variable name and brief *conceptual* definition	Source of data and *operational* definition
A. Owner:	
B. Owner:	
C. Owner:	
D. Owner:	
E. Owner:	
F. Owner:	
G. Owner:	
H. Owner:	

Side B of the Clinical Value Compass Worksheet helps in defining key operational measures for an improvement project.

Source: Reproduced with permission from The Dartmouth Institute for Health Policy and Clinical Practice (TDI).

measures of outcome and cost (Side A) and record operational definitions of those measures that are selected for actual monitoring (Side B). Users will recognize a functional connection in the compass worksheet to the Clinical Improvement Worksheet described in Chapter 3 and elaborated in Appendix A. Indeed, the two were designed for concurrent and mutually supportive use.

The Clinical Value Compass Worksheet begins with selection of a clinical population and generation of an outcomes-based aim statement to focus the improvement work. The core of the worksheet is the value compass itself. Its four cardinal points offer prompts or cues for the following categories of measurement to be considered early in the goal-defining process:

- **Clinical:** mortality and morbidity (such as signs, symptoms, treatment complications, diagnostic tests results, and laboratory determinations of physiological values)
- **Functional:** physical function, mental health, social/role function, and other measures of health status (such as pain, vitality, and perceived well-being and health risk status)
- **Satisfaction:** patient and family satisfaction with the health care delivery process, patient's perceived health benefit from care received
- **Costs:** direct medical costs (ambulatory care, inpatient services, medications, and so on) and indirect social costs (for example, days lost from work or normal routine, replacement worker costs, caregiver costs)

Using the blank Clinical Value Compass Worksheet in Figure 4-2, together with information developed on Side A of the Clinical Improvement Worksheet (*see* Chapter 3, Figure 3-1, page 24), practitioners can prepare a baseline Clinical Value Compass, map out the clinical process in question, and then construct an outcomes-based Clinical Value Compass for the "test of change" process identified.

The following initial steps will facilitate the improvement work:

1. Review (and refine, if necessary) the population and aim identified during work with the Clinical Improvement Worksheet.

2. Brainstorm ideas to generate a list of measures that are pertinent to the specified aim for each of the compass domains.
3. If working in a group setting, use multivoting or another technique to reduce this list to 4 to 12 key outcome measures.
4. Think about what data will be needed, with attention to information that can be reasonably (and affordably) obtained in real time.

The Clinical Value Compass Worksheet builds upon Russell Ackoff's advice for problem solvers: "Think up. Think down. Think up again."[12(p. 4)] Ackoff suggests that we first consider the big picture, taking the broad view before focusing on specific facets of a problem to be solved. After working on those specifics and developing a plausible solution, we then reconsider this specific solution in light of larger issues and longer-term aims. In other words, we start with strategy before going to tactics; then we check tactics and actions against strategic intent. This iterative approach is particularly useful for facilitators. The value compass worksheet might be most effective when it is not used in a linear manner, straight through from top to bottom. Instead, Side A of the value compass worksheet invites the user to "think up" and Side B to "think down."

When specific outcome variables are selected, they can be further defined both conceptually and operationally. Conceptual target outcomes might include, for example, less pain following surgery, sooner return to work after an illness episode, or greater satisfaction with the timing of a follow-up appointment. Operationally, these same variables are defined in terms of the method of measurement itself: Who collects the information and how? Thus, "pain following surgery" becomes "pain score on standardized questionnaire, administered by nurse during follow-up phone call one week after carpal tunnel surgery." All outcome variables must be similarly defined.

How is the Clinical Value Compass approach used to stimulate process improvement and to direct outcome assessment in the real world? We next review two examples in which implementation of the model is beneficial to both patients and health care organizations. We first describe in general terms one ambulatory clinic's value compass use to better understand access to primary care in the Veterans Health Administration (VHA) clinic. Then we demonstrate the specific application of the Clinical Value Compass Worksheet to improve care of patients with acute myocardial infarction in a community hospital.

Case Example: A Clinical Value Compass for Primary Care Access in VHA

In 2010 the US Veterans Health Administration (VHA) embarked on a national plan to adopt the model of the *patient-centered medical home* in an effort to improve the quality of primary care for veterans.[13] To acknowledge the contributions of many health professionals to the provision of primary care, the US Department of Veterans Affairs (VA) describes its model of the patient-centered medical home as Patient Aligned Care Teams (PACT). VHA has more than 900 sites (152 medical centers and more than 700 community-based clinics) in which the PACT model is being implemented.[14] This effort includes examining the organization of care to ensure that the health professionals needed to support each veteran are in place in every PACT.

A picture of the elements included in the PACT model is displayed in Figure 4-3, below. The model places the veteran (patient) at the center, working collaboratively with a primary care "teamlet," the exact composition of which may vary slightly, depending on the specific needs of the veteran. In general, the teamlet is composed of the primary care provider, nurse care manager, clinical associate (who is trained as a medical assistant or health technician), and clerk. This group is supported by a larger primary care team, which includes members such as administrative staff, a behavioral health

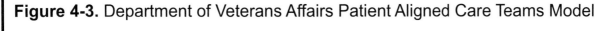

Figure 4-3. Department of Veterans Affairs Patient Aligned Care Teams Model

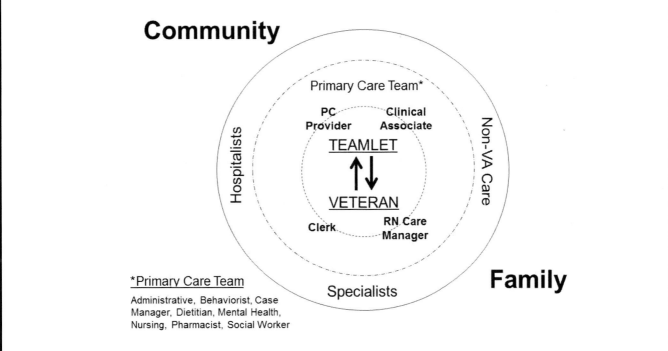

This figure provides a description of the VA's Patient Aligned Care Teams (PACT) model. The veteran and teamlet (clerk, nurse care manager, clinical associate, and primary care provider) are at the center of the model. They are surrounded by, first, the larger primary care team and, second, the larger system of hospitalists, specialists, and non-VA care.

PC: primary care; RN: registered nurse.

specialist, a case manager, a dietitian, the mental health team, nursing staff, a pharmacist, and a social worker. In addition, the primary care team works with specialists, hospitalists, and non-VA providers of care to integrate care for the veteran. The PACT model recognizes the importance of both the family of the veteran and the community in which the veteran resides.

Given the scope of the national implementation of the PACT model, VHA has devoted many resources to measuring the impact of this model on primary care specifically and care overall. VHA has defined six domains of measurement related to the PACT model:

1. Panel management
2. Patient engagement and satisfaction
3. Continuity
4. Access
5. Coordination
6. Clinical improvement

Table 4-1, below, shows the specific measures VHA is tracking in each of the six domains.

Implementation of a complex organizational intervention like PACT certainly requires multiple measures in many domains to begin to fully understand its impact. Table 4-1 lists 30 measures to track for this understanding. VHA is planning to track these measures at multiple levels of the

Table 4-1. Measures for VHA Patient Aligned Care Team implementation

Measurement Domain	Specific Measures
Panel Management	• Panel size • Panel capacity • Teamlet staff FTE • Staffing ratio • Revisit rate • Number of new patients
Patient Engagement and Satisfaction	• All-employee survey primary care satisfaction scores • Patient complaints • My HealtheVet enrollment
Continuity	• Provider: % visits with assigned primary care provider • Emergency department visit rate • Team: % visits with team
Access	• Desired date of appointment • Third next available appointment • Group clinic encounters • Telephone clinic encounters • No-show rate • Telephone access data • Secure messaging data
Coordination	• Admission rate • Patient contacted within 2 days of discharge • Patient contacted within 7 days of discharge • Consult tracking • Specialty referral rates
Clinical Improvement	• Admission rates • Emergency department visit rates • Panel case mix • Readmission rates • Ambulatory care sensitive admissions • Mortality

VHA: Veterans Health Administration; FTE: full-time employee.

organization (nationally, regionally, and locally). At the local level, one could imagine that tracking 30 measures might be quite challenging. One group in the ambulatory clinics at the White River Junction, Vermont, VA Medical Center began its work to understand the local implementation of the PACT model by focusing on the domain of access. In doing so, the clinic used the Clinical Value Compass framework as a method for reviewing a subset of the measures listed in Table 4-1. The value compass for PACT access is provided in Figure 4-4, below.

The value compass for PACT access has measures in each of the domains of clinical, functional, satisfaction, and cost. There are measures to reflect both patient and care team perspectives. The overall number of measures is fewer than in Table 4-1, which reflects the desire to focus specifically on access. Also, some of the

measures in the clinic's value compass come from domains outside of access, such as the clinical measures of diabetes, hypertension, and lipid control. These are included intentionally because the clinical team believes that improving access will improve other dimensions of primary care. Thus, the access value compass example is designed to have both core access measures and other measures that can ascertain for unintended consequences of efforts to improve access (often referred to as *balancing measures*).

In addition, Figure 4-5 (*see* Sidebar 4-1, page 46) addresses one of the key measures of access—the percentage of patients able to obtain care for the desired day of an appointment—and displays it using a statistical process control chart. The data show that before the implementation of the PACT model, 64% of veterans were able to obtain an appointment for the day desired; this process

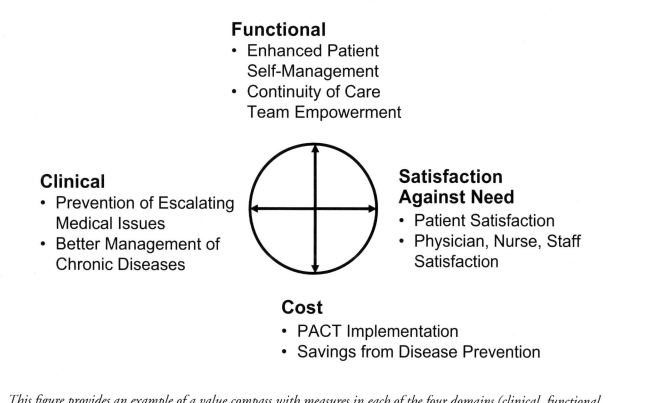

Figure 4-4. Value Compass for Department of Veterans Affairs Patient Aligned Care Team Access

Functional
- Enhanced Patient Self-Management
- Continuity of Care Team Empowerment

Clinical
- Prevention of Escalating Medical Issues
- Better Management of Chronic Diseases

Satisfaction Against Need
- Patient Satisfaction
- Physician, Nurse, Staff Satisfaction

Cost
- PACT Implementation
- Savings from Disease Prevention

This figure provides an example of a value compass with measures in each of the four domains (clinical, functional, satisfaction, and cost) related to patient-aligned care teams.

Sidebar 4-1. Primer on Statistical Process Control Charts

Health care improvement efforts require data to know that a change has resulted in an improvement.* The type of measurement and analysis used to assess any quality improvement effort should draw from both enumerative and analytic statistics.† Enumerative statistics are commonly used and include methods for assessing large databases, analysis of variance, and multivariate regression techniques, to name a few. These approaches are useful when looking retrospectively at data collected related to a quality improvement effort. Methods to analyze data prospectively over time are also useful. The most common of these analytic statistical methods is the statistical process control (SPC) chart.

SPC charts (or control charts) were first created by Walter Shewhart in the 1920s while working at Bell Labs. At that time, Shewhart was interested in creating a method for assessing the "control of quality of manufactured product" within "certain limits."‡ This approach allowed industry to replace the previous quality control methods of periodic batch inspections with ongoing assessment by frontline workers. Shewhart defined variation as coming from two types of causes:

assignable (special, nonrandom) cause and *chance* (common, random) cause. He designed the control chart to allow the user to distinguish between these causes of variation and thus take action when it is needed as well as avoid taking action when it is not needed.

There are many types of control charts available for use by health professionals seeking to improve care.§ǁ The choice of the appropriate chart is based on the type of data one is seeking to analyze. In the example shown in Figure 4-5 within this sidebar (below), we use an XmR (individuals and moving range) chart, which can be used with most types of data. The XmR chart has two components: the x-chart, which displays the actual data over time, and the moving range chart, which displays the point-to-point variation. Each chart has a center line that displays the average value for the data. The x-chart has upper and lower control limits that represent three sigma units (approximately three standard deviations) from the average. The moving range chart has only an upper control limit. For simplicity of presentation, only the x-chart is displayed in Figure 4-5, below.

There are many patterns that signify nonrandom or

Figure 4-5. Statistical Process Control Chart Example

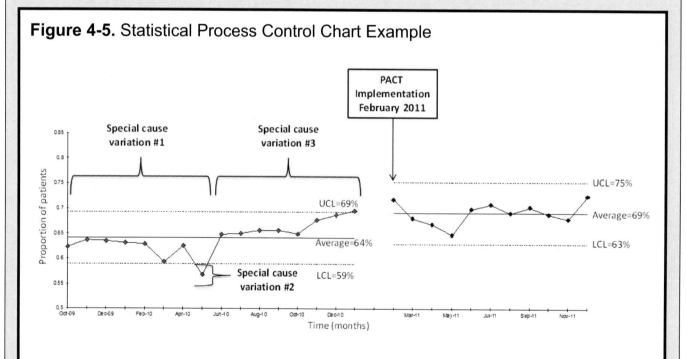

This XmR control chart illustrates the monthly proportion of VA patients seen on the desired date of appointment. The chart shows three special-cause variation signals in the initial data (October 2009 to January 2011). After implementation of patient-aligned care teams in February 2011, no special-cause signals were noted; there was no further improvement in this measure after implementation.

VA: US Department of Veterans Affairs; UCL: upper control limit; LCL: lower control limit.

Sidebar 4-1. Primer on Statistical Process Control Charts (cont'd)

assignable-cause variation. Assignable- (special-) cause variation is present if any one of the following three most common patterns is present in the *x*-chart:

1. A point above the upper control limit or below the lower control limit
2. Eight or more consecutive points above or below the center line (shift)
3. Seven or more consecutive points increasing or decreasing (trend)

If none of these patterns is present, then the variation can be considered chance (common) cause and signifies a random pattern of variation. The XmR control chart in Figure 4-5 shows average monthly proportion of primary care patients seen on the desired date of appointment at the White River Junction Veterans Affairs primary care clinics before and after Patient Aligned Care Team (PACT) implementation in February 2011. The data are displayed over 26 months. The data from the first 16 months show an average of 64%. In addition, the data reveal three special-cause signals (downward shift noted as special-cause variation #1, point below the lower control limit noted as special-cause variation

#2, and upward shift noted as special-cause variation #3). The average and control limits were split at the time of the intervention of PACT, as this represents a different process for access to primary care than prior to the intervention. After PACT implementation, the data for proportion of patients seen on the desired day of appointment show an average of 69% and no special-cause signals; thus, there is only common-cause variation present. The process is in statistical control.

References

* Langley GL, et al. *The Improvement Guide: A Practical Approach to Enhancing Organizational Performance,* 2nd ed. San Francisco: Jossey-Bass, 2009.

† Provost LP. Analytical studies: A framework for quality improvement design and analysis. *BMJ Qual Saf.* 2011 Apr;20 Suppl 1:i92–96.

‡ Shewhart WA. *Economic Control of Quality of Manufactured Product.* 1931. Milwaukee: ASQ Quality Press, 1980.

§ Amin SG. Control charts 101: A guide to health care applications. *Qual Manag Health Care.* 2001;9(3):1–27.

‖ Carey RG. *Improving Healthcare with Control Charts: Basic and Advanced SPC Methods and Case Studies.* Milwaukee: ASQ Quality Press, 2003.

---

was highly variable and not predictable. Since implementation of the PACT model, an average of 69% of veterans are able to have an appointment for the day desired; this process is less variable and more predictable. Although this represents an improvement, the clinic team recognizes that the goal of "excellent" access has not yet been achieved. Thus, the team's work to continue to improve the processes of care and monitor the results is ongoing.

This first example of the Clinical Value Compass approach demonstrates the use of the framework as a method for focusing the work of practice-based learning and improvement of a small set of measures that inform the work in multiple domains. The second example that follows provides a more detailed description of the use of the Clinical Value Compass framework in making improvement in the care of patients—in the case of acute myocardial infarction.

Case Example: A Clinical Value Compass for Acute Myocardial Infarction

Acute myocardial infarction (AMI) remains a leading cause of morbidity and mortality for American adults and a common reason for emergency room presentation and hospital admission. Although timely delivery of evidence-based interventions has been shown to reduce the incidence of adverse outcomes, such interventions are not delivered consistently across all emergency departments and hospitals.[15,16] The Clinical Value Compass Worksheet supports exploration and improvement of value-based health care services. Here, we invite the reader to join a clinical improvement team endeavoring to optimize AMI care at a local community hospital. Accompanying figures demonstrate specific use of the value compass worksheet in this case.

Side A—Getting Started: Outcomes and Aim

The process begins with a statement of aim linked to desired outcomes for a target population. This is an invitation to "think up" strategically. The aim statement answers the question, "What are we trying to accomplish?"[17(p. 24),18] In this case, as shown in Figure 4-6 (page 50), the team selects an AMI population for observation over a certain time period: patients with confirmed AMI who are directly admitted to the hospital (that is, nontransfer patients). The clinical process starts when the patients are admitted to the emergency department and ends eight weeks after they have been discharged.

The team selects a clinical population and time period for which the clinical team has primary responsibility for patient care. Next, the team clarifies its aim and writes down its answer to the questions, "Given our desire to limit or reduce the burden of illness for AMI patients, what are the desired results? What's the aim?" The team describes its aim: to find ways to continually improve the quality and value of care for AMI patients.

Although a general aim statement (as just presented) is usually the best place to start, over time most teams will revise the statement to more precisely capture the true aim. The increased specificity results from the following:

- Description of the current clinical care process
- Identification of potential changes that are expected to lead to improvement
- Selection of specific high-leverage changes to test using a PDSA (Plan–Do–Study–Act) cycle

When designing a value compass, the clinical team can envision important measures of outcome and cost by "circling the compass" in clockwise rotation—that is, by beginning with clinical status and proceeding to functional status, satisfaction, and costs. Subcategories of measures are bulleted under each of the Clinical Value Compass axes, reminding users of the types of variables that might be considered under each broad area. Knowledge of the appropriate clinical literature is essential, though its utility is greatly facilitated by complementary knowledge of daily experiences in local patient care. Different team members might bring expertise in different domains. Considered in combination, this diverse base of knowledge and experience will yield a large number of potential measures. Decision-making skills—such as brainstorming to generate ideas and multivoting to reduce the long list to a manageable number of measures—can be very helpful as well.[19]

Note that the Clinical Value Compass Worksheet begins with questions that aim to capture clinical professionals' ethical values. Given our desire to limit

or reduce the illness burden for this type of patient, what are the desired results? What is the aim? The patient remains at the value compass's center and focuses work explicitly on the ethical canon of the healing professions—on the ongoing search for better ways to improve patient care.

A word of caution: Although the list of potential outcome measures can be long, we advise value compass worksheet users to focus initial efforts on a relatively small number of key measures so that reasonably accurate information can be collected at an affordable cost. Remember, our intention is to improve our ability to characterize the results of care from the perspective of value. As a rule of thumb, 4 to 12 carefully chosen outcome measures are sufficient to get started. Because we often lack any systematically available measures for clinicians' performance, a "developmental" approach to measurement is appropriate. Begin data collection on a small scale: More measures can be added as time passes, as experience is gained, and as information requirements evolve.

This list summarizes the starter set of measures selected by the team for initial monitoring of all AMI patients:

1. Clinical status
   - Death in hospital or within eight weeks after discharge
   - Angina symptoms
2. Functional status
   - Physical function
   - Overall health
3. Satisfaction against need
   - Patient satisfaction with hospital
   - Change in overall health
4. Costs
   - Total hospital charges
   - Length of stay in hospital
   - Days lost from work or normal routine

The clinical team used nominal group methods and brainstorming to produce a long list of potential measures of outcomes; it then used multivoting to reduce this list to a smaller, more manageable number of measures for which data could be gathered from one of three sources:

1. Medical record review
2. Administrative and billing data

3. Patient-based data gathered by mailed questionnaire (with telephone follow-up of nonrespondents) at eight weeks after discharge

Although the list of outcomes is small, the team did define one or more measures for each of the four value compass quadrants, assuring a "balanced" approach to data collection and quality assessment.

Side B—Operational Definitions of Measures

Side B of the Clinical Value Compass Worksheet provides space to record "think down" tactical ideas in the form of specific definitions for key measures of outcome or cost. For each measure, participants create both a conceptual definition (brief description of the dimension or phenomenon of interest) and a precise operational definition (specific, reliable, and understandable process that translates the concept into a reproducible observation on each patient). If the operational definition is based on a previously published or validated measure, the source can be listed on the value compass worksheet as well. Figure 4-6 (page 50) provides definitions for most of the measures selected by the AMI team. Precision and clarity are essential in the statement of the operational definitions.[20] Additional examples of measures with associated operational definitions for AMI care have been published by Spertus et al.[21] Reliability and validity of measures are critically dependent on clear and consistent application of these definitions. The measures themselves will be extracted from data in the medical record, administrative and financial records, and patient reports and ratings at eight weeks after discharge.

When plans for specific Clinical Value Compass measures have been clarified and recorded on the value compass worksheet, the next steps involve designing the following[22]:

- A data collection plan (consider using a simple chart or illustration that describes who, what, where, when, and how for each measure)
- An analysis plan to answer important questions
- A method to display information and distribute results
- Use of the results for managing patients and improving care

Displays might include graphic depictions of both summary information (for example, results for the first 50 patients) and comparative information (results for this quarter versus a previous quarter; or results of this organization versus another organization). Control charts might be used for individual outcomes or costs, revealing variations and trends over time (a control chart showing length of stay for the past 24 months). A trial or "dummy display" of measures can be helpful. The clinical process instrument panel in Figure 4-7 (page 51) connects process measurements to discrete steps in the delivery of AMI care. Value compass–based outcome results for the project are summarized in Figure 4-8 (page 51).

Advice on the Worksheet Approach

We at The Dartmouth Institute for Health Policy and Clinical Practice have used the Clinical Value Compass approach and the Clinical Improvement Worksheet since 1995, and, on the basis of our experience, we offer the following suggestions for their combined use.

Be Flexible. The overall aim is to accelerate clinical improvement, not to slavishly follow any one method for making these improvements. There are two flaws to avoid when making improvements: going too fast and going too slow. Individual clinicians and larger clinical teams might sometimes benefit from proceeding quickly through Side A of the Clinical Value Compass Worksheet and from skipping the construction of precise definitions (Side B) until a specific test of change has been selected. Often, in the case of team-based work, the very occasion of coming together to discuss a common patient care problem will yield many ideas for improvement. In these situations, there can be value in performing a test of change that all participants agree is worthwhile, even if they do not agree on its relative priority. We often underestimate how much we can learn from the manner in which the system "pushes back" when we try to change it.

When a test of change has been selected, operational definitions can be created for key outcome measures specific to this intervention. These measures can then be tracked in real time at

Figure 4-6. AMI Clinical Value Compass Worksheet, Side A

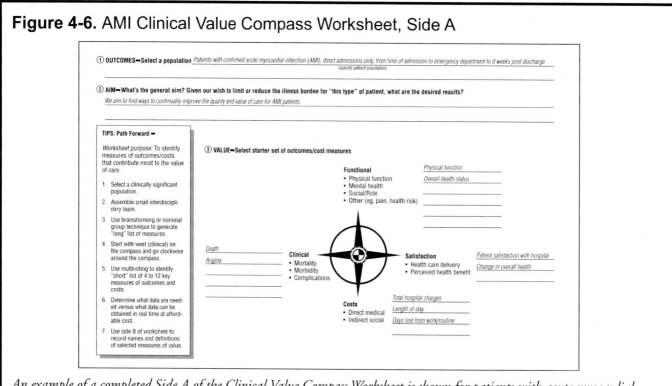

An example of a completed Side A of the Clinical Value Compass Worksheet is shown for patients with acute myocardial infarction (AMI).

Source: Reproduced with permission from The Dartmouth Institute for Health Policy and Clinical Practice (TDI).

Figure 4-6. AMI Clinical Value Compass Worksheet, Side B

④ SPECIFIC OPERATIONAL DEFINITIONS → for key outcome and cost measures

TIPS: Writing Definitions →	Variable name and brief *conceptual* definition	Source of data and *operational* definition
A *conceptual definition* is a brief statement describing a variable of interest. It should tell people **what** you want to measure and who "owns" it. An *operational definition* is a clearly specified **method** for reliably sorting, classifying, or measuring a variable. It should be written as an instruction set, or protocol, that would enable two different people to measure the variable by using the same process and thereby producing the same result. It should explain to people **how** a variable should be measured.	A. *Death:* patient dies during hospital stay or within 8 weeks postdischarge. Owner: _____	*Medical record* review indicates patient died, or *follow-up* by mail/telephone at 8 weeks indicates patient died.
	B. *Angina:* angina pectoris—pain in chest associated with coronary artery disease (Rose scale). Owner: _____	*Patient's* answers to four questions at 8 weeks coded to form scale: 27. Do you ever have any pain or discomfort in your chest? ❑ Yes ❑ No 28. If no, do you ever have any pressure or heaviness in your chest? ❑ Yes ❑ No 36. Do you have this pain, discomfort, pressure, or heaviness when you walk uphill or hurry? ❑ Yes ❑ No 37. Do you have these symptoms at an ordinary pace on level ground? ❑ Yes ❑ No
	C. *Physical function:* the ability to perform physical activities associated with normal living (COOP scale). Owner: _____	*Patient's* answer to one question at 8 weeks: 26. During the past 2 weeks, what was the most strenuous level of physical activity you could do for at least 2 minutes? ❑ Very heavy, eg,_____ ❑ Heavy, eg,_____ ❑ Moderate, eg,_____ ❑ Light, eg,_____ ❑ Very light, eg,_____
	D. *Overall health:* patient's general perception of his/her health status (COOP scale). Owner: _____	*Patient's* answer to one question at 8 weeks: 1. During the past 2 weeks, how would you rate your overall physical health and emotional condition? ❑ Excellent ❑ Very good ❑ Good ❑ Fair ❑ Poor
	E. *Patient satisfaction with hospital:* patient's overall rating of inpatient care and services (HQT item). Owner: _____	*Patient's* answer to one question at 8 weeks: 33. How likely would you be to return to this hospital if you ever needed to be hospitalized again? ❑ I'm 100% sure that I'd return. ❑ I probably would not return. ❑ It's very likely that I'd return. ❑ It's very unlikely that I'd return. ❑ I probably would return. ❑ I'm 100% sure that I would not return. ❑ I'm not sure if I would return. ❑ Does not apply to me because I do not live near hospital.
	F. *Change in overall health:* patient's perception of the health benefit received from care. Owner: _____	*Patient's* answer to one question at 8 weeks: 7. Overall, is your health better or worse than you expected it to be at this point? ❑ Much better than I expected ❑ Somewhat worse than I expected ❑ Somewhat better than I expected ❑ Much worse than I expected ❑ About what I expected
	G. *Total hospital charges:* the sum of all inpatient charges to the patient for the stay, excluding physician charges. Owner: _____	Search of hospital's *billing records* to determine total sum of charges billed to the patient's account for the hospital stay.
	H. *Length of stay:* number of days patient stayed in hospital. Owner: _____	*Medical record* review used to determine date of admission and date of discharge; length of stay computed based on interval.

An example of a completed Side B of the Clinical Value Compass Worksheet is shown for patients with acute myocardial infarction (AMI).

Source: Reproduced with permission from The Dartmouth Institute for Health Policy and Clinical Practice (TDI).

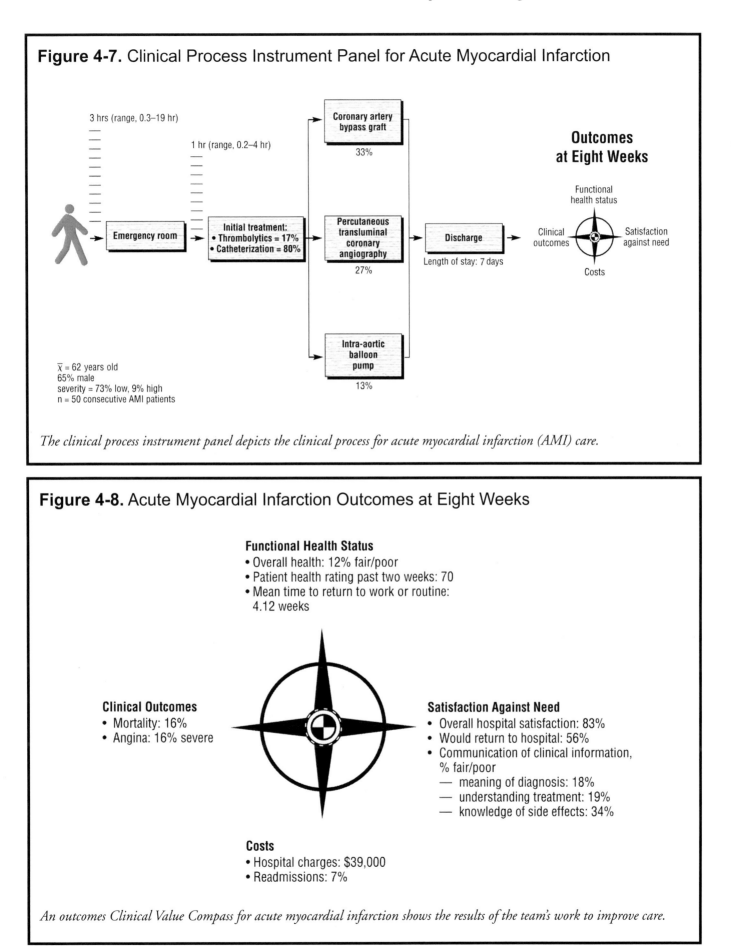

Figure 4-7. Clinical Process Instrument Panel for Acute Myocardial Infarction

3 hrs (range, 0.3–19 hr)

1 hr (range, 0.2–4 hr)

Emergency room

Initial treatment:
• Thrombolytics = 17%
• Catheterization = 80%

Coronary artery bypass graft
33%

Percutaneous transluminal coronary angiography
27%

Intra-aortic balloon pump
13%

Discharge
Length of stay: 7 days

Outcomes at Eight Weeks

Functional health status

Clinical outcomes

Satisfaction against need

Costs

$\overline{x}$ = 62 years old
65% male
severity = 73% low, 9% high
n = 50 consecutive AMI patients

The clinical process instrument panel depicts the clinical process for acute myocardial infarction (AMI) care.

Figure 4-8. Acute Myocardial Infarction Outcomes at Eight Weeks

Functional Health Status
• Overall health: 12% fair/poor
• Patient health rating past two weeks: 70
• Mean time to return to work or routine:
  4.12 weeks

Clinical Outcomes
• Mortality: 16%
• Angina: 16% severe

Satisfaction Against Need
• Overall hospital satisfaction: 83%
• Would return to hospital: 56%
• Communication of clinical information,
  % fair/poor
  — meaning of diagnosis: 18%
  — understanding treatment: 19%
  — knowledge of side effects: 34%

Costs
• Hospital charges: $39,000
• Readmissions: 7%

An outcomes Clinical Value Compass for acute myocardial infarction shows the results of the team's work to improve care.

an affordable cost. If a clinician or clinical group is committed to long-term improvement and repeated tests of change, then a value compass–based data set can be wisely developed that gathers and analyzes information continuously, permitting clinicians to spot favorable trends, to monitor progress, and to quickly detect adverse events.

Start Small. The Clinical Value Compass approach reminds us that quality and value are multidimensional. Practitioners might feel overwhelmed by the large number of potential variables and might therefore feel tempted to measure everything from the start. This is generally a mistake. The wiser initial strategy is to select a small, balanced set of important outcome measures, chosen because they can be measured reasonably well and because they "hit" each of the four Clinical Value Compass quadrants. New and better measures can be added at any point in the future.

Build Measurement into the Delivery Process. Measurement systems that quantify the quality of patient care are too frequently added on to routine care delivery after the fact. Although this approach permits customized design and standardization, it also adds new costs (in terms of time, labor, and material resources) and thus might reduce actual value. To enhance efficiency and effectiveness, measurement should be built into the care delivery process itself. For example, in an emergency department with an electronic health record (EHR) in which an improvement team is trying to understand waits and delays in the process from check-in to being seen by a clinical provider, it would be advisable to use the electronic time stamps in the EHR to assess the time rather than ask each member of the process to write down the time that he or she interacted with the patient. The latter approach adds the work of collecting data to the job of providing care. The former approach makes use of the existing system for data collection and does not add work to those providing care. Incorporating data collection without adding work allows frontline providers to be engaged in both management of the patient and measurement of processes and related outcomes. The new measures can be used in real time to improve care for the individual patient, and they can be immediately

accessed to facilitate redesign of care for future patients.[23] Improvement teams must therefore select measures that can be implemented by those involved in service provision itself and that drive the desired quality characteristic of the result.

Use Measurement Instruments Already Available in the Clinical Improvement Literature. Practitioners do not need to "reinvent the wheel" when devising measurement schemes for parameters of clinical interest. Many simple and validated instruments are publicly or commercially available and can be incorporated into clinical practice with little or no modification. In Appendix C (pages 153–154) we have collected examples of and Web links to several such instruments. We invite the reader to adapt these forms to local caregiver contexts. Further material can be downloaded from a number of useful websites of organizations focusing on the improvement of quality and patient safety, some of which are listed in Appendix E (pages 159–161).

Recognize Limitations. Although the value compass approach enables users to analyze the value of health care and identify targets for improvement, several limitations must be noted. First, the Clinical Value Compass does not generate prospective information about patient preferences, nor does it identify excess capacity in the system. Second, unless the approach is supplemented by appropriate control charts that document variation over time, important signals cannot be separated from random noise. (Refer to Sidebar 4-1 on pages 46–47.) Third, pursuit of the most rigorous and advanced Clinical Value Compass applications requires mastery of several measurement methodologies (including measurement of clinical outcomes, functional status and well-being, patient satisfaction with care, cost accounting, and financial burden of illness assessment), as well as application of formal analytic techniques (such as summation of rating scales, risk adjustment/stratification, and cost-effectiveness analysis). The availability of validated measurement instruments (such as those provided in Appendix C) simplifies the measurement process somewhat but does not eliminate the need for sophistication in data collection and analysis.

The Clinical Value Compass can be used in the

real world in a more or less sophisticated manner, depending on needs, circumstances, available resources, level of experience, and technical knowledge. Many users have found the Clinical Value Compass framework to be the following:

- Useful in providing a logical and balanced framework for measuring and improving care
- Appealing to diverse stakeholders—physicians, nurses, patients, purchasers, and planners
- Flexible and robust across a variety of caregiving contexts

Clinical Value Compass Complements Strategies to Improve Organizational Performance

We have emphasized throughout this chapter the utility of value compass thinking in identifying patient-oriented outcomes and improvement strategies. The Clinical Value Compass concept can be used to complement frameworks such as the balanced scorecard that help leaders guide organizational performance. To be successful in today's health care environment, organizations should to be able to address two fundamental questions:

1. Is the system providing care and services that meet patients' needs for high-quality and value-based care?
2. Is the organization performing in a way that will enable it to grow and survive, given available resources?

The Clinical Value Compass framework can be used to address the first question. The balanced scorecard can be used to address the second question. The value compass approach combines both clinical and patient-reported data (Figure 4-9, below). These data are represented in multiple domains to provide the best possible understanding

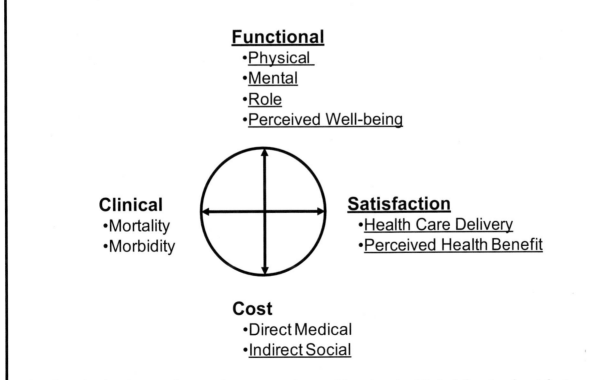

Figure 4-9. Clinical Value Compass Framework Combining Clinical and Patient-Reported Data

Functional
- Physical
- Mental
- Role
- Perceived Well-being

Clinical
- Mortality
- Morbidity

Satisfaction
- Health Care Delivery
- Perceived Health Benefit

Cost
- Direct Medical
- Indirect Social

The Clinical Value Compass framework encourages the use of four domains (clinical, functional, satisfaction, cost) to describe the health status of an individual or a population for a given condition. The figure provides examples of generic measures for each domain and emphasizes that measures can be collected from the clinician perspective as well as from patient-reported measures (underlined).

of the health status of an individual or a population of patients. The data can be assessed at a single point in time or can be monitored over time to observe for changes in health status. The focus or unit of analysis for the value compass is the patient or population of patients being served. This focus distinguishes the value compass from the balanced scorecard, which focuses on the organization or specific unit within an organization.

Clinician and nonclinician leaders of health care organizations often use a balanced scorecard of measures to address the second question by assessing systemwide performance in strategic and business domains. This popular approach was developed and refined by Kaplan and Norton[24,25] for use in manufacturing sectors, but it has been widely adopted (and adapted) by service organizations in general (and by health systems in particular) in the United States and around the world. The balanced scorecard makes use of four perspectives:

1. **Innovation and Learning.** What must we learn and how must we innovate to be successful in meeting the needs of patients, families, staff, and other beneficiaries? What can we learn from others and from the competitive environment about better ways to meet these needs? What services and products need to be developed, and what processes require innovation?

2. **Core Processes.** What actions and activities need to work efficiently, reliably, and accurately to provide needed services and products? How can we streamline and error-proof our processes? How can we reduce real costs while improving quality, efficiency, and beneficiaries' perceptions?

3. **Beneficiaries' Perceptions.** How are we perceived by the (external and internal) beneficiaries of our essential services? How do we compare, in terms of these perceptions, to our direct and indirect competitors? What do beneficiaries expect, want, and need? What delights them, and what disappoints them? What prompts defections, and what contributes to loyalty? What attracts individuals to our organization, and what attracts them to our competitors?

4. **Finance and Growth.** How do our economics look to our shareholders and to our board? Are volumes and revenues growing as planned and needed? Are unnecessary costs being removed without sacrificing technical and service quality? Are we making sufficient margins to build and secure our future? Are human resource assets growing as needed, and where needed, or are we losing human capital in mission-critical areas?

The unit of analysis for the balanced scorecard is the part of an organization (microsystem or mesosystem) providing care to a population of patients.

The complementary nature of the value compass and balanced scorecard is shown in Figure 4-10 (page 55). The figure depicts a simplified schematic of a clinical microsystem.[26] The microsystem serves a population of patients with an initial burden of illness prior to receiving care. Care provided by health professionals in the microsystem results in outcomes that ideally are a new lesser burden of illness. The value compass provides an organized approach to measuring the outcomes of care for the population served by the microsystem. The balanced scorecard provides an approach to assessing the results of the microsystem's performance overall.

Concluding Thoughts

In this chapter, we described the Clinical Value Compass framework as an approach to understanding the value of care provided to an individual or a population of patients. We provided two examples of the use of the value compass—one in primary care related to access and the other in specialty care related to cardiac services for patients with myocardial infarction. Finally, we offered an approach to understanding organizational improvement by combining the value compass with the balanced scorecard. We hope the reader can appreciate the many ways in which the Clinical Value Compass framework can be used or adapted to guide the improvement of care.

In Chapter 5, we build on this foundation by extending our thinking from what we are currently

Figure 4-10. Complementary Nature of Clinical Value Compass and Balanced Scorecard

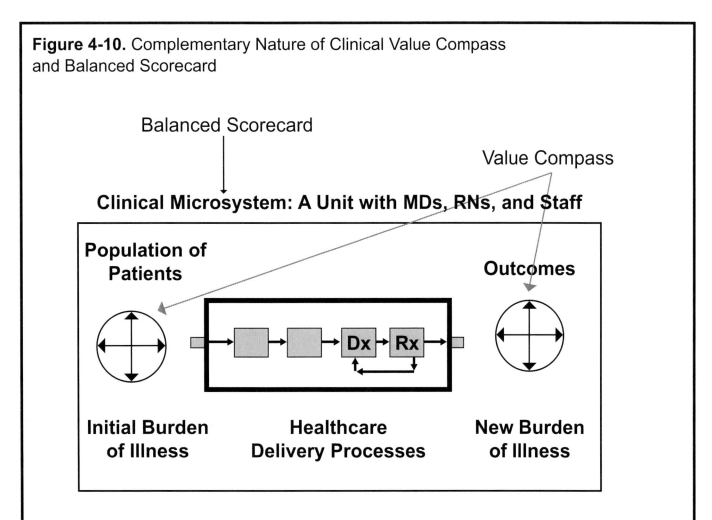

A clinical microsystem (large box) is defined as a unit with health professionals and staff who serve a population of patients through health care delivery processes (small boxes). The Clinical Value Compass is useful for describing the burden of illness for the population served by the microsystems; the unit of analysis is an individual or a population of patients. The burden of illness can be described over time as represented in the figure—initial burden and new burden of illness after receiving care in the microsystem. The balanced scorecard is useful for assessing system performance in strategic and business domains; the unit of analysis is the microsystem.

achieving to what we could possibly achieve through benchmarking—understanding the best of the best and the process for becoming so.

Acknowledgement

The authors wish to thank the following graduate students from The Dartmouth Institute for Health Policy and Clinical Practice who contributed to the project described in this chapter related to VA PACT implementation during their graduate studies: Danielle M. Crochiere, MPH; Alecsa Mackinnon Blair, MPH; and Rima S. Shah, MPH.

References

1. Zapato Productions Intradimensional. Lord Kelvin (Sir William Thomson): "Quotations." (Updated: Dec 14, 2008.) Accessed Oct 16, 2012. http://zapatopi.net/kelvin/quotes/.

2. Rosenthal MB, et al. Early experience with pay-for-performance: From concept to practice. *JAMA.* 2005 Oct 12;294(14):1788–1793.

3. Personal communication between the author [E.C.N.] and Stephen K. Plume, MD, President, Lahey Hitchcock Clinic, and Professor, Department of Surgery, Dartmouth Medical School, Lebanon, NH, 1996.

4. Porter ME, Olmstead Teisberg E. *Redefining Health Care: Creating Value-Based Competition on Results.* Boston: Harvard Business School Press, 2006.

5. Committee on Redesigning Health Insurance Performance Measures, Payment, and Performance Improvement Programs,

Institute of Medicine. *Performance Measurement: Accelerating Improvement.* Washington DC: National Academies Press, 2006.

6. Womack JP, Jones DT, Roos D. *The Machine That Changed the World.* New York: HarperCollins, 1991.

7. Dubos RJ. *The Mirage of Health: Utopias, Progress, and Biological Change.* New York: Doubleday Anchor, 1961.

8. Rice DP, Feldman JL, White KL. *The Current Burden of Illness in the United States.* Washington, DC: Institute of Medicine, National Academy of Sciences, 1976.

9. Susser M. Health as a human right: An epidemiologist's perspective on the public health. *Am J Public Health.* 1993 Mar;83(3):418–426.

10. World Health Organization (WHO). Constitution of the World Health Organization. In WHO, *Basic Documents,* 47th ed. Geneva: WHO, 2010, 1–18.

11. Donabedian A. *Explorations in Quality Assessment and Monitoring,* Vol. 1, *The Definition of Quality and Approaches to Its Assessment.* Ann Arbor, MI: Health Administration Press, 1980.

12. Ackoff RL. *The Second Industrial Revolution.* Herndon, VA: Alban Institute, 1975.

13. Commonwealth Fund. The Veterans Health Administration: Implementing Patient-Centered Medical Homes in the Nation's Largest Integrated Delivery System. Case Study: High-Performing Health Care Organization. Klein S. Sep 2011. Accessed Oct 17, 2012. http://www.commonwealthfund.org/~/media/Files/Publications/Case%20Study/2011/Sep/1537_Klein_veterans_hlt_admin_case%20study.pdf.

14. US Department of Veterans Affairs. Patient Aligned Care Teams (PACT) Demonstration Lab Initiative: Research-Clinical Partnerships to Evaluate and Enhance VA PACT Implementation. Yano B, et al. Feb 17, 2011. Accessed Oct 17, 2012. http://www.visn4.va.gov/VISN4/CEPACT/HSRD_2011_DemoLab.pdf.

15. McGlynn EA, et al. The quality of health care delivered to adults in the United States. *N Engl J Med.* 2006 Jun 26;348(26):2635–2645.

16. Peterson ED, et al. Association between hospital process performance and outcomes among patients with acute coronary syndromes. *JAMA.* 2006 Apr 26;295(16):1912–1920.

17. Langley GJ, et al. *The Improvement Guide: A Practical Approach to Enhancing Organizational Performance,* 2nd ed. San Francisco: Jossey-Bass, 2009.

18. Langley GJ, Nolan KM, Nolan TW. The foundation of improvement. *Quality Progress.* 1994 Jun;27(6):81–86.

19. Scholtes PR, Joiner BL, Streibel BJ. *The Team Handbook,* 3rd ed. Madison, WI: Oriel, 2003.

20. Deming WE. *Out of the Crisis.* Cambridge, MA: Massachusetts Institute of Technology Center for Advanced Engineering Study, 1986.

21. Spertus JA, et al. American College of Cardiology and American Heart Association methodology for the selection and creation of performance measures for quantifying the quality of cardiovascular care. *Circulation.* 2005 Apr 5;111(13):1703–1712.

22. Nelson EC, Batalden PB. Patient-based quality measurement systems. *Qual Manag Health Care.* 1993;2(1):18–30.

23. Nelson EC, et al. Microsystems in health care: Part 2. Creating a rich information environment. *Jt Comm J Qual Saf.* 2003 Jan;29(1):5–15.

24. Kaplan RS, Norton DP. *The Balanced Scorecard: Translating Strategy into Action.* Boston: Harvard Business School Press, 1996.

25. Kaplan RS, Norton DP. *Strategy Maps: Converting Intangible Assets into Tangible Outcomes.* Boston: Harvard Business School Press, 2004.

26. Nelson EC, Batalden PB, Godfrey MM, editors. *Quality by Design: A Clinical Microsystems Approach.* San Francisco: Jossey-Bass, 2007.

Chapter 5

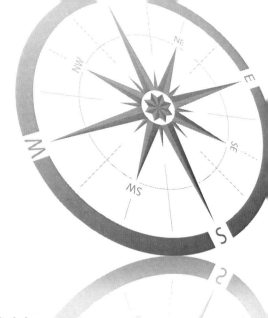

Learning from the Best: Clinical Benchmarking for Best Patient Care

Justin Glasgow, Carlos A. Estrada, Tracy Shamburger, Mark E. Splaine, Julie K. Johnson, Eugene C. Nelson, Paul B. Batalden, Peter Kaboli

There is always one best result and one best process for achieving that result ... and they can always be improved.

—Brian Joiner[1]

Why has benchmarking created such interest in health care? Increased competition, significant practice variation, and the need for better communication of variation in outcomes and costs are some of the reasons for increased attention to benchmarking.[2] Benchmarking allows a committed practitioner to learn what works best and to define goals for improvement on the basis of what is known.

Practice-based learning and improvement requires that we not only reflect on our own clinical and administrative processes but also compare with peers to identify and possibly implement best practices. Such comparison can inspire and direct our own work. Clinical benchmarking empowers us to identify and to implement "best practices" that we had not previously considered—nor even thought possible. An important outcome from the benchmarking process is the learning that occurs in terms of one's own processes, not merely adopting some other organization's successful practices. The microsystems of care described in Chapter 1 are unique to each organization; hence, solutions for one organization need to fit into the larger system. The following quotations from an infection control collaborative highlight the potential influence of benchmarking:

In our network of hospitals, 10 hospitals have some of the lowest central catheter–related infections. What can we learn from what they do?

I just attended our annual meeting on public health departments. Small health departments similar to ours are achieving the best influenza and pneumococcal immunization rates in their areas. I did not think that was possible.

In this chapter we introduce a process for clinical benchmarking that facilitates the identification and implementation of best health care practices. The benchmarking process builds on the foundations for improvement and targeting interventions (Chapters 1 and 2) and makes use of the Clinical Improvement Worksheet and the Clinical Value Compass (Chapters 3 and 4, respectively). The reader would benefit from reviewing prior chapters or could start with this one if a process has already been implemented and data are available.

We review basic benchmarking concepts and offer a benchmarking worksheet to further guide improvement efforts. We briefly review the evidence and practical applications of audit and feedback as they relate to benchmarking. We describe the ABC™ method to compute benchmarks—Achievable Benchmarks of Care—a methodology that is objective, reproducible, and attainable to measure and analyze performance on process-of-care indicators.[3] Finally, we review concrete examples from health care on how the benchmarking process has been embedded in practical applications. We invite readers to adapt benchmarking methods to improvement work in their own context.

Benchmarking and Its Use in Health Care

Benchmarking in health care has been adapted from other settings and industries, where well-established definitions are available. The concept is derived from the Japanese industrial practice *dantotsu*, which refers to a method for finding the "best of the best"—the best practice that consistently produces best-in-the-world results.[4] The concept was developed after World War II and spread rapidly throughout the United States and the industrial world. Xerox Corporation pioneered the formal methodology of *benchmarking* in the 1980s, defining it as "the continuous process of measuring [the company's] products, services, and practices against [its] toughest competitors or those companies known as leaders."[4] In the 1990s Camp and Tweet simplified this definition to "finding and implementing best practices."[5(p. 230)]

Benchmarking and benchmarks are different concepts, although sometimes the terms are mistakenly used interchangeably. The design of effective improvement strategies depends on appropriate use of the two ideas, which are defined as follows:

- *Benchmarking:* a systematic process of searching to identify best practices
- *Benchmark:* a statistical measure of the results of a given practice

When the benchmarking *process* is performed without consideration of statistical benchmark *measures*, the specific merits of various practices are not fully evaluated. Conversely, if only benchmarks are assessed, no insight is gained into the actual process identified as best practice. In both industry and health care, advocates of improvement often forge ahead prematurely, armed with benchmarks but lacking an understanding of the underlying processes that produced them.

When benchmarking techniques are used effectively and combined with appropriate analysis of resulting statistical measures (the benchmarks), the overall process can stimulate local improvement. Benchmarking processes bring the following interdependent benefits:

- Create tension for change
- Build awareness of current local capability versus best-known capability anywhere
- Encourage people to move from a position of inertia to one of positive action
- Foster diverse ways of thinking about the conduct of the care/work

An awareness of performance variation between sites challenges reflective practitioners to ask why the variation exists. The appreciation of alternate solutions contributes to the tension for change and motivates professionals to work individually and collectively.

For some organizations, an early step in the benchmarking process is to identify peers or partners or competitors to benchmark against. Building such relationships, in the case of peers or partners, enables participants to compare outcomes of interest but also fosters an appreciation of underlying processes and structures of care. This comparison can prove beneficial for both the group seeking and the group providing the benchmark. Such collaboration can have both short- and long-term benefits for each group. Because benchmarking against a single organization may not provide "best of the best" benchmark measures, it is important to reach beyond the most readily available benchmark. Two complementary approaches to benchmarking include the use of local and national benchmarks (for example, other hospitals or health systems) and evidence-based practices documented in the literature. Benchmarking is not always successful. Poor planning, lack of institutional support, lack of ownership, insufficient skills, and perceived low priority are some factors associated with unsuccessful processes.

In this chapter, we focus on benchmarking techniques[6] specifically to improve important clinical processes to reduce illness burden and to improve value in patient care. Important administrative processes such as billing, payroll, and supply management chain can also benefit from the benchmarking process we describe; however, they are beyond the scope of this chapter, as excellent benchmarking partners exist in other industries.

Benchmarking and the Clinical Improvement Worksheet

In Chapter 3 we presented the Clinical Improvement Worksheet to incorporate improvement work in busy clinical practices. As shown in Figure 3-1 (pages 24–25), the worksheet provides a template for improvement for a specific test of change. Briefly, the following questions are used to guide the improvement process:

- What is the general aim of this work, and whom are we trying to help?
- What is the process for giving care to this type of patient?
- What ideas do we have for changing what is done (the process) to get better results?

- How can we pilot test an improvement idea?
- Who should work on this improvement?
- What are we trying to accomplish?
- How will we know whether a change is an improvement?
- How would we describe the change that we have selected for testing?
- How shall we plan the pilot?
- What are we learning as we do the pilot?
- As we study what happened, what have we learned?
- As we act to hold the gains or abandon our pilot efforts, what needs to be done?

Benchmarking and the Clinical Value Compass

Chapter 4 described the Clinical Value Compass, which can guide the benchmarking process. As shown again in Figure 5-1 (below), the cardinal points in the compass define the domains that matter to patients, providers, and other stakeholders, delineating important outcomes most worthy of benchmarking investigation: clinical

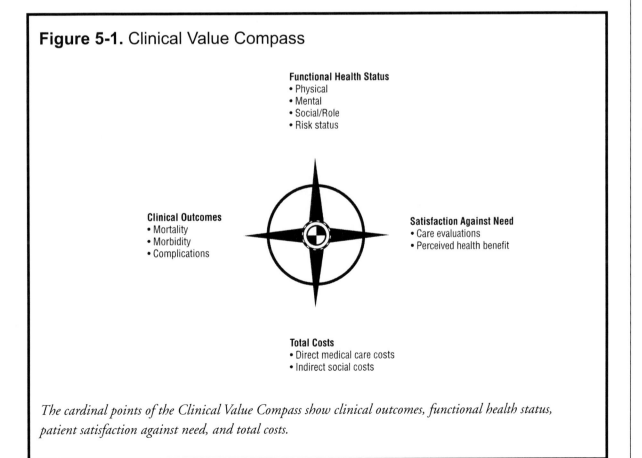

Figure 5-1. Clinical Value Compass

Functional Health Status
- Physical
- Mental
- Social/Role
- Risk status

Clinical Outcomes
- Mortality
- Morbidity
- Complications

Satisfaction Against Need
- Care evaluations
- Perceived health benefit

Total Costs
- Direct medical care costs
- Indirect social costs

The cardinal points of the Clinical Value Compass show clinical outcomes, functional health status, patient satisfaction against need, and total costs.

outcomes, functional health status, satisfaction against need, and total costs.[7] Initially, the charges paid can serve as markers of cost; however, indirect costs must be considered as well because the goal is to identify ways to minimize the economic burden of illness.

Benchmarking for Best Practices: A Planning Worksheet

Various models have been described for benchmarking, including Motorola (5 steps), AT&T (9 steps), and Xerox (10 steps).[8] The distinctions among the various models are not as important as their similarities; all successful processes share several common features. Each reflects a systematic, measured approach to benchmarking that follows a basic format—plan, collect, analyze, and improve.[8]

Building on the Clinical Improvement Worksheet and the Clinical Value Compass, we present a two-sided modified worksheet for benchmarking purposes, as shown in Figure 5-2 (pages 61–62). Like other tools presented in this book, the benchmarking worksheet was designed to guide the improvement process, record results, and document the process. The specific aim of the benchmarking process is to develop testable ideas about best practices. The benchmarking worksheet divides the process into the following five basic steps:

1. Identify statistical measures (benchmarks).
2. Determine resources needed to find the best of the best.
3. Design the data collection method and gather data.
4. Measure best against own performance to determine performance gaps.
5. Identify the best practices that produce best-in-class results.

Step 1. Identify Statistical Measures (Benchmarks)

Step 1 defines the statistical measures (that is, benchmarks) that will focus the search outside one's own setting for best practices (also called external scan). Using the Clinical Value Compass as a guide, practitioners define the two or three measures for clinical outcomes, functional health status, satisfaction against need, and total costs. Generally, many measures are identified early in the improvement process. During or after the implementation for the clinical improvement work (Chapters 1–4), planning and implementing a benchmarking process could be done in parallel or in sequence. Reducing the number of measures during this process will simplify the search and comparison. Figure 5-2, Side A, provides space for documenting and summarizing the key aspects of the tasks to be completed.

We recommend focusing on a few key measures that do the following:
- Allow measurement and comparison across facilities or locations
- Reflect variability of performance across facilities or locations
- Serve as valid comparison data
- Represent the important outcomes of care

Step 2. Determine Resources Needed to Find the Best of the Best

Step 2 defines the resources to generate and summarize the best data, identify the best people to perform the benchmarking process, and retrieve the best available literature. Internal and external data need to be as accurate as possible to ensure that comparisons are valid and reliable. Internal data might need to be reformatted to allow comparison with external sources. The measures identified in the first step can be used as keywords to focus the literature search. Benchmarking teams would benefit from creating and summarizing a bibliography of relevant articles if none is available. Step 2 also involves secondary research—querying available sources to maximize knowledge on a given subject. This step may not necessarily reveal the actual processes that best-of-the-best clinical sites use to achieve their results. Providers who offer such benchmark outcomes are usually willing to share their insights into care processes linked to their outcome measures. Valuable people resources include a range of stakeholders who are local leaders and experts most familiar with the clinical process, the data, and the techniques of benchmarking and improvement processes. Local experts can also

Figure 5-2. Benchmarking for Best Practices, Side A

Aim: Develop ideas about best practices.

1. Identify measures.

Using the Clinical Value Compass as a guide, reach a consensus on 2 or 3 statistical measures, or benchmarks, that will be the focus of the external scan. Consider the availability of valid comparative data and variability of performance across facilities. (An appropriate benchmark enables measurement and comparison across systems.)

Functional Health Status

Clinical Outcomes

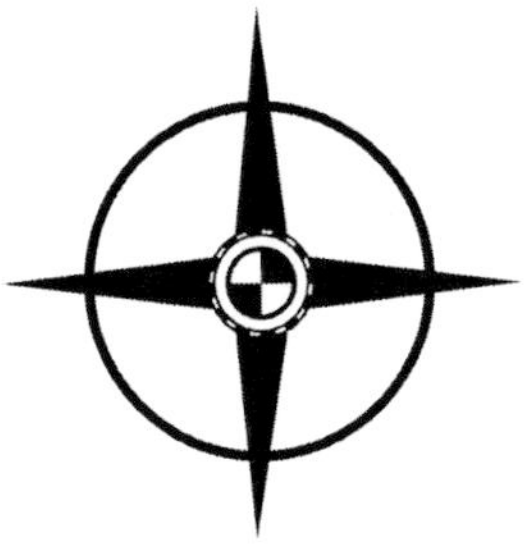

Satisfaction Against Need

Total Costs

2. Determine resources needed to find the best of the best.

Given our desire to limit or reduce the illness burden (cost, resource use, excess morbidity, mortality) for our patients, think about the information needed for finding the best of the best.

The best data to use? Internal? External?	The best people to ask? In-house? Out-of-house?

The best literature?

Side A of the benchmarking worksheet helps develop ideas about best practices by completing secondary research to identify measures and needed resources.

Reproduced with permission from The Dartmouth Institute for Health Policy and Clinical Practice (TDI).

Figure 5-2. Benchmarking for Best Practices, Side B

3. **Design data collection method and gather data.**
   Who will collect the data? How will the data be analyzed? Who will review the literature?

   Task: **Person completing:**   **Date to be completed:**

   _____

   _____

   _____

   _____

   _____

   _____

4. **Measure best against own performance to determine gap.**
   Based on the measures identified in step 1, and the results of an internal and external scan of the data, how does our performance compare to the best of the best?

   Benchmark: _____

Our results	_____
Average	_____
"Best"	_____

   Benchmark: _____

Our results	_____
Average	_____
"Best"	_____

Summary Data	
Number of cases:	_____
Total revenue:	_____
Revenue rank:	_____

   Benchmark: _____

Our results	_____
Average	_____
"Best"	_____

   Functional Health Status

   Clinical Outcomes — Satisfaction Against Need

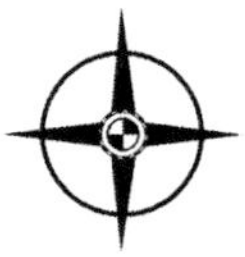

   Total Costs

   Compared to what we found, how good is our quality and value?

   Benchmark: _____

Our results	_____
Average	_____
"Best"	_____

   Benchmark: _____

Our results	_____
Average	_____
"Best"	_____

   Benchmark: _____

Our results	_____
Average	_____
"Best"	_____

5. **Identify the best practices that produce best-in-class results.**

Side B of the benchmarking worksheet organizes data collection tasks and records performance.

identify external experts. A rich source for obtaining information is based on the network of personal contacts and interactions at professional societies or meetings.

Large health care delivery systems, such as the US Department of Veterans Affairs (VA) and Kaiser Permanente (*see* Chapter 8 for examples) have developed the infrastructure to share measures of best practices. In addition, QualityNet, established by the Centers for Medicare & Medicaid Services (CMS), provides resources and data reporting tools and applications for participating institutions to compare performance measures.[9] The Joint Commission also annually publishes the list *Top Performers on Key Quality Measures,*™ which could be mined for benchmarking.[10]

Step 3. Design the Data Collection Method and Gather Data

Step 3 helps the team establish a method and time line for data collection and analysis. The process thus gains focus and is kept on schedule. Figure 5-2, Side B, also provides space for documenting and summarizing the key aspects of the data collection tasks to be completed, the individuals who will complete them, and the time line. For example, identifying the statistical measures and benchmarks (Step 1) requires a team member to commit to research those measures in a timely manner. Similarly, completing the remaining tasks illustrated in Figure 5-2, Side B, requires an explicit approach to assign responsibilities.

Step 4. Measure Best Against Own Performance to Determine Performance Gaps

During Step 4, the team compares its own results with external measures and best practices. Tension for change is generated when a performance gap is recognized between internal performance and best-practice performance. The value to define a clinically important gap is usually defined by the problem itself and by the team within the context of the organization. The benchmarking worksheet in Figure 5-2 provides space for internal results, national average results, and the best of the best. To provide a broader context, space is also provided

to record summary data for number of cases, total revenue, and revenue rank. For an organization, the revenue rank is the rank for the total revenue generated by the specific problem to be addressed. For example, a high-volume activity that generates significant revenue is ranked higher than a low-volume, low-revenue-generating activity.

Step 5. Identify the Best Practices That Produce Best-in-Class Results

In Step 5, the team identifies processes that produce best results to close the performance gap. The work performed thus far supports participants' understanding of relationships between processes and outcomes. As mentioned at the start of this chapter, perhaps the most important outcome from the benchmarking process is the learning that occurs by examining one's own processes. Tension for change is recognized, and specific improvement ideas are generated. The organization can identify potential benchmarking partners and establish a mutually beneficial learning relationship.

It is important to optimally understand internal processes and clearly assess external information before potential benchmarking partners are contacted. This knowledge base will make time spent with benchmarking partners more efficient because detailed understanding will sharpen subsequent questions and improvement interventions.

It is at this point that the team can use the Clinical Improvement Worksheet (described in Chapter 3) to plan another rapid cycle for improvement. Parallel processes occur between internal analysis of one's own organization (guided by the Clinical Improvement Worksheet) and external assessment of similar organizations (for example, of practice sites that serve similar patient populations). The results of this initial benchmarking work then feed back into the Clinical Improvement Worksheet to stimulate additional ideas for change.

From Benchmarking to Clinical Care

The work described thus far enables practitioners and larger organizations to clarify their own processes and experiences and compare them with benchmarking partners or with exemplary practices and use the literature to identify best-of-the-best results. Health care organizations can use data from benchmarking work to partner effectively with other sites toward a shared goal of optimizing patient care at all sites.[11] Benchmarking partnerships have the potential to enable participating organizations to share best practices that are at the heart of their own performance and to learn from best practices performed elsewhere. An excellent example is the Greater New York Hospital Association's central line–associated bloodstream infection (CLABSI) collaborative. During the 33-month collaborative, CLABSI rates dropped by 54% ($p < .001$) and were sustained after the collaborative ended.[12]

However, we offer a cautionary note: Pfeffer and Sutton identified "casual" benchmarking, in which well-intentioned efforts fail because organizations approach collaborative learning in a casual instead of systematic way.[7] Casual benchmarking is ineffective because the focus is on copying the most visible and obvious practices, even though these might also be the least important practices.[8] Also, as outlined by Mark Chassin, president of The Joint Commission, "the most fundamental reason that best practices don't work the same way everywhere is that they were developed to work on a different set of causes than the ones you have at your organization."[13(p. 475)]

Audit and Feedback

The benchmarking process can be used to provide feedback to the practitioner, team, or health systems. Again, the feedback provided also creates tension for improvement. The process of audit and feedback is a well-established method in quality improvement.

An updated Cochrane review of 118 studies synthesizing the best available evidence showed that well-developed feedback can be effective in improving patient care.[14] The magnitude of the benefit, however, is small, and feedback delivered in a more intensive fashion yields better results. The magnitude of the improvement is also higher when performance levels are low. The review concludes: "Providing healthcare professionals with data about their performance (audit and feedback) may help improve their practice. Audit and feedback can

improve professional practice, but the effects are variable. When it is effective, the effects are generally small to moderate. The results of this review do not support mandatory or unevaluated use of audit and feedback as an intervention to change practice."[14]

Audit and feedback has been implemented in the VA using External Peer Review Program (EPRP) rankings to guide improvement interventions.[15,16] For example, in one study, EPRP was used to compare high-performing versus low-performing facilities.[17] In a systematic review in nursing, a model using audit and feedback has been suggested to improve cancer pain control.[18] Furthermore, audit and feedback has been used to improve catheter-associated asymptomatic bacteriuria.[19]

Finally, in graduate medical education, audit with or without formal feedback has also been associated with improved processes of care.[20] Audit and feedback is a method that meets the practice-based learning and improvement core competency requirement for graduate medical education residency programs and is included in the practice-based learning general competency requirement of the American Board of Medical Specialties for maintenance of certification.[21,22]

Selecting a Measure and a Benchmark

Ideal performance indicators are valid, reliable, and sensitive to change. A recent review summarized additional characteristics: Ideal measures of performance should also be communicable, objective, available and feasible, contextual, attributable, interpretable, comparable, actionable, repeatable, adaptable, acceptable, and relevant to policy.[23] However, such characteristics are often not encountered in routine performance measures. Hence, defining the most suitable ones requires a balance between perfection (highly accurate) and the opportunity cost that is required to be clinically applicable.

An *accountability measure* is a measure that is used (usually by others) for public reporting, payment, or regulation. All accountability measures should meet criteria for benchmarking for improvement measures, but not all benchmarking for improvement measures need to meet all the criteria to be accountability measures. The Joint Commission has defined *accountability measures* as quality measures that meet four criteria that produce the greatest positive impact on patient outcomes when hospitals demonstrate improvement. Chassin and colleagues described these four criteria for accountability measures that address process of care as follows[24]:

1. There is a strong evidence base showing that the care process leads to improved outcomes.
2. The measure accurately captures whether the evidence-based care process has, in fact, been provided.
3. The measure addresses a process that has few intervening care processes that must occur before the improved outcome is realized.
4. Implementing the measure has little or no chance of inducing unintended adverse consequences.

The *Top Performers on Key Quality Measures*™ program uses a specific evidence-based methodology to identify and recognize hospitals that attain and sustain excellence. The program includes certain conditions such as heart attack, heart failure, pneumonia, surgical care, and children's asthma.[10]

An important aspect to consider is that in some settings, best practices still fall short of the desired performance. An example of this scenario is hand washing in health care settings. Although hand washing has been recognized as a low-cost intervention to prevent nosocomial transmission, hand-washing rates remain in the 40% range.[25,26]

Benchmarks must represent a measurable level of excellence and also should be demonstrably attainable. Furthermore, providers with high performance (and without exclusion) should be selected from all providers in a predefined manner based on an objective measurement of actual performance. Providers with high performance but with a relatively small numbers of cases should not unduly influence the benchmark level. The ABC method meets these criteria. Funded by the Agency for Healthcare Research and Quality (AHRQ), the ABC methodology is an objective, reproducible, attainable approach to measure and analyze performance on process-of-care indicators.[27,28]

The theoretical framing of the method may seem complicated, but the computation of benchmarks is mathematically simple. A step-by-step manual is available in the public domain.[3] In essence, the achievable benchmark represents the average performance for the top 10% of the practitioners being assessed.

Although the ABC methodology was initially designed to identify the top 10%, the applicability for such an approach has been demonstrated by rigorous studies. For example, randomized controlled trials using the ABC methodology in quality improvement projects have shown exciting results in some studies,[29–32] but not all.[33] In the setting of a multimodal quality improvement intervention, for example, implementing the ABC methodology as feedback to the practices was associated with improved diabetes process measures performance (influenza immunization, foot exam, laboratory testing).[29] Similarly, in a multifaceted improvement intervention among physicians in training in two specialties—internal medicine and pediatrics—receipt of preventive services in their respective patient groups remained unchanged in the control group and increased in the intervention group (for adults in internal medicine: smoking screening, quit smoking advice, colon cancer screening, pneumonia vaccine, and lipid screening; for pediatrics: parental quit smoking advice, car seats, car restraints, and eye alignment).[32] The multifaceted feedback curriculum included individualized performance feedback (using ABC methodology), academic detailing, and didactic sessions.

Benchmarking in Health Care: Selected Experiences

In the following selected experiences in health care, we illustrate how peer comparison and benchmarking are applied to improve patient care, quality, and safety. To illustrate the range of possibilities of the use of benchmarking, we present a process improvement project for hospital discharge documentation (Sidebar 5-1, pages 66–67), a response to a national and statewide mandate for surgical site infections (Sidebar 5-2, pages 68–69), and international efforts in population health (Sidebar 5-3, page 69). The

Sidebar 5-1. Case Study: Benchmarking for Best Practices, Hospital Discharge Documentation

At the request of the chief of medicine, a quality improvement team was established on the inpatient medical service at the Iowa City Veterans Affairs (VA) Health Care System in Iowa City, Iowa, in the fall of 2010 to improve the timeliness of discharge summary completion. The baseline standard at the hospital was for completion of a discharge summary within 48 hours of discharge, yet for 10% to 15% of the discharges, a summary was not completed within seven days of discharge. This created potential patient safety concerns (for example, the discharge summary is the primary source of communication between inpatient and outpatient providers), reduced patient satisfaction (patients are unhappy when their primary care providers are unaware of follow-up needs or miss test results), affected hospital operation (delays in documentation and billing, extra work to monitor and remind physicians to complete the summaries), and could lead to violation of Joint Commission standards. Table 5-1 (page 67) summarizes the five steps of the quality improvement team's benchmarking and improvement process.

This example represents a simple approach to benchmarking. The measures were quickly agreed upon, the data were readily available and understandable (such as the delinquency rate), best-of-the-best processes were already known, and measuring progress was easily performed monthly to assess impact.

Step 1: Identify Statistical Measures (Benchmarks)
The project began with a pair of internal medicine physicians working to evaluate the discharge process and the documentation related to discharge at the hospital. Guided by the Clinical Value Compass, the team, led by a hospitalist, worked to identify potentially relevant measures of the process. Some examples of measures included rate of delinquent discharge summaries (functional), patient and provider satisfaction (satisfaction), readmission rates (clinical), and administrative time spent tracking discharge summaries (costs). After reviewing the list of brainstormed measures, the team decided to focus primarily on the rate of delinquent discharge summaries. Some strengths of this measure were that historical data were available and that it was a direct process measure that was likely to reflect improvements. The team also decided to monitor patient satisfaction scores and query primary care providers about their satisfaction with the documentation throughout the process.

Step 2: Determine Resources Needed to Find the Best of the Best
After the initial background work, the next step was to bring together a team capable of providing or accessing the critical knowledge and experience needed to ensure a thorough and successful improvement project. The final team comprised inpatient and outpatient physicians, inpatient and outpatient pharmacists, a nurse manager, staff from the quality and compliance offices, the chief of medicine, and, in the later stages of the project, a programmer for the electronic medical record. This team met to review the list of statistical measures, confirmed the decision to focus on delinquency rates, and began to think about how to obtain information from the literature and other institutions to determine the best current practices.

Step 3: Design the Data Collection Method and Gather Data
During this stage, the team worked to modify current data collection processes at the hospital to provide optimal information related to delinquent discharges. For local data collection, the team focused on obtaining additional details about delinquent discharges, such as level of physician responsible for the delay (resident or attending) and potential sources of special-cause variation (for example, patients leaving against medical advice). To inform the improvement process and provide baseline data, the team developed a six-question survey for primary care providers and inpatient resident physicians. To query outside resources, the team developed a strategy for querying relevant Listservs and the academic literature to obtain details about other approaches to discharge documentation.

Step 4: Measure Best Against Own Performance to Determine Gap
Initial local data collection at the facility confirmed the historical rates of delinquent discharges with a mean rate of delinquent discharge summaries at 11%. This was in comparison to a variety of approaches that produced a 0% delinquency rate at other academic institutions by ensuring that discharge summaries were not only completed prior to discharge but also were provided directly to the patient at discharge. Although the hospital provided discharge instructions, several elements of the discharge summary were not currently provided directly to patients.

continued on next page

Sidebar 5-1. Case Study: Benchmarking for Best Practices, Hospital Discharge Documentation, *continued*

Step 5: Identify the Best Practices That Produce Best-in-Class Results

In a six-month period, the team worked to bring together critical features from discharge summaries at their local academic affiliate, other VA hospitals, and other quality improvement efforts such as the Society of Hospital Medicine's Project BOOST (Better Outcomes for Older adults through Safe Transitions) to develop a single document that providers could complete before discharge without delaying discharge.

The key to success was identifying steps in the process and realizing that providers were already completing written discharge instructions, a task required prior to patient discharge. By incorporating the discharge instructions with the discharge summary into one simplified yet inclusive document, providers were able to complete the discharge summary prior to discharge without additional work. In fact, the new process simplified the discharge process by removing a step: creating a separate discharge summary after discharge.

A number of Plan–Do–Study–Act (PDSA) cycles were carried out, and the new discharge template was rolled out gradually to providers to allow adjustments of the format. The template was rapidly and voluntarily adopted by providers, with a reduction in discharge delinquencies to 0% after eight months of implementation.

In this example, it happened that a peer institution had adopted a system that worked well to address a common problem. Because neither the process nor the improvement steps were complex, the level of benchmarking required for more complex systems was unnecessary. The benchmarking partnership described has the potential to enable participating organizations to share best practices that are at the heart of their own performance and to learn from best practices performed elsewhere.

Not all benchmarking and improvement teams work as well as this one, but this case study illustrates how identifying small but important areas for improvement can result in "early wins" for improvement teams and gives them the confidence and skills to attack more complex problems—such as medication reconciliation and prevention of errors—in the future.

Table 5-1. Benchmarking for Best Practices, Hospital Discharge Documentation

Step 1. Identify Statistical Measures (Benchmarks)	Discharge summary completed: within 72 hours (peer hospital), within 24 hours (hospital policy), or before discharge (best of the best) Discharge summary provided to patient at discharge (best of the best) Immediate availability of discharge summary to primary care provider (satisfaction) Rapid preparation of third-party billing (costs)
Step 2. Determine Resources Needed to Find the Best of the Best	Best data: number of discharge summaries delinquent past 24 hours Best people to ask: peer institutions within Veterans Affairs (VA) health care system; non-VA hospitals; hospitalist quality improvement network Best literature: limited information
Step 3. Design the Data Collection Method and Gather Data	Monthly historical data on discharge summary delinquencies for the past year at hospital for internal medicine service Administrative officer for service to distribute
Step 4. Measure Best Against Own Performance to Determine Gap	Monthly rate of discharge summary delinquency greater than 24 hours Best practice: 0% (all discharge summaries completed prior to discharge) Our baseline rate: 12-month average of delinquent discharge summaries: 11%
Step 5. Identify the Best Practices That Produce Best-in-Class Results	The university hospital academic affiliate where physicians from the VA also practiced had adopted a policy requiring discharge summaries to be completed prior to discharge, resulting in a 0% delinquency rate.

Sidebar 5-2. Case Study: Benchmarking in a State Initiative on Surgical Site Infections

In July 2010 a 300-bed hospital in Alabama sought to improve the surveillance of surgical site infections (SSIs) using the National Healthcare Safety Network (NHSN) of the US Centers for Disease Control and Prevention (CDC).*[†]

Two external forces facilitated the process: the US Centers for Medicare & Medicaid Services (CMS) reporting mandate of SSIs[‡] within the next two years and a new state mandate requiring a monthly report of abdominal hysterectomies and colon surgeries. The number of procedures and SSIs would be reported from all hospitals within the state to the public within 12 months of the mandatory reporting period. Both required the use of the NHSN definitions. In addition, internal patient care issues were important to lower SSI rates (including SSIs not requiring hospital readmission) and the high financial burden.

Like the organization profiled in Sidebar 5-1, the Alabama hospital in this case study followed a five-step process of benchmarking.

Step 1: Identify Statistical Measures (Benchmarks)
The NHSN criteria for SSI patients undergoing abdominal hysterectomies and colon surgeries served as the statistical data or benchmark in this scenario (as shown in Table 5-2, below).

Step 2: Determine Resources Needed to Find the Best of the Best
The resources were identified to meet the benchmark. The team/group was composed of a physician leader, a nurse, and infection control specialists. However, the team continued to collect data on amount of time required, number of personnel, accuracy, and delays

in reimbursement of the manual data collection and reporting. In addition, the need for random internal validation of cases reported was identified.

Step 3: Design the Data Collection Method and Gather Data
The team conferred with other peers through the Association for Professionals in Infection Control and Epidemiology (APIC).[§] Although multiple measures were identified, the team quickly noted a need to prioritize the benchmarking actions on the basis of available resources and the immediate time constraints. First, the team noted the lack of a reference standard for postdischarge surveillance for SSIs and the variance of postdischarge practices among hospitals within the state. To ensure meaningful comparisons, the Alabama Department of Public Health convened a group of statewide stakeholders to develop a set of minimum postdischarge surveillance standards. Hence, the local team focused on the immediate concerns—timely and accurate identification and reporting of procedures and SSIs using the NHSN.

Six months before the monthly mandatory reporting of SSI data was to begin, the team reviewed the current steps employed in identifying patients who underwent the selected surgical procedures. International Classification of Diagnosis-9 (ICD-9) codes were not deemed appropriate because their assignment was often delayed beyond 30 days. The team decided to report the procedure description independent of ICD-9 coding. Surgical nurses were educated on collecting NHSN–relevant data for the selected surgeries (for example, length of the procedure) to the infection control practitioners electronically each day. After the ICD-9

Table 5-2. Benchmarking a State Initiative—Surgical Site Infections (SSIs)

Step 1. Identify Statistical Measures (Benchmarks)	US Centers for Disease Control and Prevention's National Healthcare Safety Network (NHSN) criteria for SSIs Patients undergoing abdominal hysterectomies and colon surgeries
Step 2. Determine Resources Needed to Find the Best of the Best	Best people to ask: peer institutions, Association for Professionals in Infection Control and Epidemiology (APIC)
Step 3. Design the Data Collection Method and Gather Data	Daily identification of patients Infection control nurse
Step 4. Measure Best Against Own Performance to Determine Gap	Monthly SSI rates for selected surgeries In development; public reporting was due to begin after July 2012.
Step 5. Identify the Best Practices That Produce Best-in-Class Results	In development; public reporting was due to begin after July 2012.

continued on next page

Sidebar 5-2. Case Study: Benchmarking in a State Initiative on Surgical Site Infections, *continued*

codes were available, edits to the data were made as needed. The team also identified resources needed for data collection.

Step 4: Measure Best Against Own Performance to Determine Gap
As of January 2011, the surgical procedures were reported monthly on time in the NHSN. Data edits or missing information after audits were minimal. The public reporting was due to begin after July 2012.

Step 5: Identify the Best Practices That Produce Best-in-Class Results
This step had not been implemented at the time of this writing because follow-up data from the public reporting were not yet available.

References
* Centers for Disease Control and Prevention. National Healthcare Safety Network (NHSN). (Updated: Sep 18, 2012.) Accessed Oct 17, 2012. http://www.cdc.gov/nhsn/index.html.
† Centers for Disease Control and Prevention. CDC/NHSN Surveillance Definition of Healthcare-Associated Infection and Criteria for Specific Types of Infections in the Acute Care Setting. Jan 2012. Accessed Oct 17, 2012. http://www.cdc.gov/nhsn/PDFs/pscManual/17pscNosInfDef_current.pdf.
‡ Centers for Medicare & Medicaid Services. Medicaid program; payment adjustment for provider-preventable conditions including health care-acquired conditions. Final rule. *Fed Regist.* 2011 Jun 6;76(108):32816–32838.
§ Association for Professionals in Infection Control and Epidemiology, Inc. (APIC). Home Page. Accessed Oct 17, 2012. http://www.apic.org.

Sidebar 5-3. Benchmarking in International Health

International benchmarking of quality of care may help motivate improvement. Significant efforts are under way to develop and validate quality and safety performance measures. As mentioned in Step 2 of the benchmarking process (page 60), valid and reliable data enable comparison with local or regional practices.

In the United Kingdom, the National Quality Board (NQB) is charged with overseeing quality indicators and examining international benchmarks for quality and safety improvement. A RAND Corporation report reviewed three National Health Service priorities: effectiveness of care, patient safety, and patient experience.* Much as according to the sequence described earlier in the benchmarking worksheet (pages 61–62), NQB is to provide a summary of the methods and measures for quality indicators (process or outcome measures), review the literature, and assess suitability of existing indicators for comparison. As compared to clinical outcomes, process indicators are more sensitive to change, are easily measured, enable detection of changes earlier, and reflect aspects of care important for patients and stakeholders.

When conducting benchmarking, organizations might consider comparison of performance according to the following:
- World Health Organization Health Systems Performance Assessment Framework focuses on health system performance (health, responsiveness, equity).
- Organisation for Economic Co-operation and Development Health Care Quality Indicators project focuses on technical quality of health care (effectiveness, safety, responsiveness, patient-centered).
- Dutch Health Care Performance Report focuses on quality, access, and costs.
- National Scorecard on US Health System Performance (US National Scorecard) focuses on performance on specific benchmarks.

Examples of quality indicators of effectiveness of care for international comparison and benchmarking include vaccinations (for example, measles, hepatitis B), cancer care (mammography screening, survival), cardiovascular care (acute myocardial infarction readmissions), respiratory diseases (asthma mortality), diabetes care (retinal exam, HbA1c testing), and children's health (infant mortality). Other examples exist for patient safety and patient experience. International efforts are under way for comparing and benchmarking quality of care, patient safety, and patient experience indicators.

Reference
* Nolte E. *International Benchmarking of Healthcare Quality: A Review of the Literature.* Santa Monica, CA: RAND Corp., 2010. Accessed Nov 26, 2012. http://www.rand.org/pubs/technical_reports/TR738.html.

teamwork and collaboration at a large academic medical center example shown in Chapter 8 (Sidebar 8-1, pages 98–99) illustrates various steps of the benchmarking process described in this chapter.

Infection Control

Health care–associated infections (HAIs) account for significant morbidity, mortality, and costs. In one review, the author notes opportunities by using "bundles" of interventions (rather than single interventions) to decrease infections.[34] Also, to change the culture, the author proposes a "zero tolerance approach" instead of the traditional benchmarking. Finally, a culture of accountability and administrative support is required. Infection control areas proposed by the Institute for Healthcare Improvement (IHI) include prevention of central line–associated bloodstream infection, surgical site infection, ventilator-associated pneumonia, and methicillin-resistant *Staphylococcus aureus* (MRSA) infection. Those areas of infection control, as well as prevention of influenza and catheter-associated urinary tract infections, are addressed by The Joint Commission's HAI Portal, a website full of related resources (http://www.jointcommission.org/hai.aspx).

Surgical Care

The World Alliance for Patient Safety at the World Health Organization (WHO) compiled and disseminated a manual to implement the Surgical Safety Checklist.[35] The checklist identifies three phases of a surgical intervention: before anesthesia induction ("Sign In"), before skin incision ("Time Out"), and before the patient leaves the operating room ("Sign Out"). The manual provides suggestions for implementation, considering each local environment. Messahel and Al-Qahtani provide a formal assessment of the use of the checklist.[36]

Beginning in 2013, hospitals and ambulatory surgery centers will be expected to annually report to CMS whether staff used a safe surgery checklist during the prior year. Although CMS does not require the use of a specific checklist, it provides examples of checklists, including the WHO Surgical Safety Checklist and The Joint Commission's

Universal Protocol for Preventing Wrong Site, Wrong Procedure, Wrong Person Surgery™.[37] A reporting tool and further information are available on the QualityNet website.[9]

Patient Safety Attitudes

Investigators at the University of Texas examined the validity (psychometric properties) of a safety attitudes questionnaire.[38] During the international process in 203 clinical areas (including critical care units, operating rooms, inpatient settings, and ambulatory clinics), they also established benchmarks. The main components of the safety attitudes questionnaire included teamwork climate, safety climate, perceptions of management, job satisfaction, working conditions, and stress recognition. Institutions can use the instrument for benchmarking and to foster interventions to enhance patient safety.

Collaboration Initiatives

Although not specifically a benchmarking process, collaborative initiatives, as fostered by IHI, The Joint Commission, and other organizations, include benchmarking processes—namely, developing a learning network (develop teams), identifying best practices (compare across practices), data audit (design data collection method and gather data), and feedback.

A collaborative approach and campaigns have been used in patients with AIDS to increase rates of highly active antiretroviral treatment initiation in South Africa,[39] decrease MRSA infections,[40] reduce fall injuries among hospitalized patients,[41] and decrease readmissions.[42]

Summary Remarks

The health care environment continues to grow increasingly transparent to clinical providers, patients, and other purchasers. With quality and cost data more available for public scrutiny, benchmarking knowledge and benchmark data are increasingly easy to obtain. Thus, appropriate use of comparative measurements can be used to identify best-practice organizations and stimulate wise clinical changes and demonstrable improvements in quality and value. Benchmarking can locate areas of improvement in the broader health care context and will be addressed in future chapters that reconsider the process of change in both individuals and institutions.

The following principles can serve as a guide to benchmarking:

- *Someone, somewhere is best.* Although it might not be a single provider, someone, somewhere does practice in a way that produces the best results in clinical outcomes, functional status, satisfaction, and costs. Learning about best practices is the aim of benchmarking. Yet even "the best" are not necessarily the ideal. Moreover, benchmarking does not always consider context-specific factors, such as local practice variation, access to services, population demographics, and payer characteristics. A truly optimal health system must include continual improvement of the processes of care, continual assessment of current treatments, and identification and reallocation of excess capacity. Such a system is usually somewhere beyond both current performance and existing best-known practices.
- *Benchmarking is (just) a tool.* Although benchmarking is a useful tool for identifying and learning about best practices, it is just one step in the journey toward optimal health care delivery.
- *Benchmarking can create tension for change.* Benchmarking goes beyond the mere replication of what others are doing to achieve similar outcomes. Benchmarking could lead to changes and to implementation of innovative activities.
- *Benchmarking is an ongoing process involving everyone.* Benchmarking helps clinicians continually assess the external environment and leads to best practices and outcomes. Clinical improvement is the job of everybody, whether individual practitioners or loosely or highly organized work groups or teams. The process of benchmarking is particularly conducive to collaborative interactions. Effective benchmarking teams combine the clinical experiences of frontline practitioners and staff with the analytic, quantitative, and qualitative

skills of data and benchmarking coordinators.
- *Benchmarking requires leadership, process knowledge, and commitment.* Although the leader of benchmarking activities need not be a practicing clinician, this individual will benefit from familiarity with the processes of patient care and from a regular working relationship with the clinical staff. Indeed, Camp and Tweet emphasize the importance of all team members being actively involved in the work of their own benchmarking: "When the process owners conduct their own benchmarking, they develop a commitment to the process and the resulting best practices."[5](p. 237) Finally, both concerted management support and carefully designed communication are essential for all effective benchmarking processes.

In this chapter, we reviewed the process for clinical benchmarking that will help organizations reflect on their own practice, identify gaps, explore opportunities for improvement, and learn from the best performers. The next chapter explores underlying change concepts that support the generation and elaboration of specific improvement ideas—in particular, resistance and readiness for change and models to implement change.

References

1. Joiner B. Reflections on Dr. Deming's contributions to management. Closing keynote address at the Eighth Annual International Deming User's Group Conference. Paper presented at Ohio Quality and Productivity Forum, Aug 17, 1994.
2. Wennberg JE, et al. *The Dartmouth Atlas of Health Care.* Chicago: American Hospital Publishing, 1996.
3. University of Alabama at Birmingham (UAB). Achievable Benchmarks of Care (ABC™) User Manual. Weissman N, et al.; UAB Center for Outcomes and Effectiveness Research. 1999. (Updated: Sep 20, 2001.) Accessed Oct 17, 2012. http://main.uab.edu/show.asp?durki=11311.
4. Camp RC. *Business Process Benchmarking: Finding and Implementing Best Practices.* Milwaukee: ASQC Quality Press, 1995.
5. Camp RC, Tweet AG. Benchmarking applied to health care. *Jt Comm J Qual Improv.* 1994 May;20(5):229–238.
6. Campbell AB. Benchmarking: A performance intervention tool. *Jt Comm J Qual Improv.* 1994 May;20(5):225–228.
7. Pfeffer J, Sutton RI. *Hard Facts, Dangerous Half-Truths, and Total Nonsense: Profiting from Evidence-Based Management.* Boston: Harvard Business Press, 2006.
8. American Productivity and Quality Center (APQC). *The Benchmarking Management Guide.* Cambridge, MA: APQC, 1993.

9. QualityNet. Home Page. Accessed Oct 17, 2012. https://www.qualitynet.org.

10. The Joint Commission. Top Performers on Key Quality Measures.™ Accessed Oct 17, 2012. http://www.jointcommission.org/accreditation/top_performers.aspx.

11. Sharek PJ, et al. Best practice implementation: Lessons learned from 20 partnerships. *Jt Comm J Qual Patient Saf.* 2007 Dec;33(12 Suppl):16–26.

12. Koll BS, et al. The CLABs collaborative: A regionwide effort to improve the quality of care in hospitals. *Jt Comm J Qual Patient Saf.* 2008 Dec;34(12):713–723.

13. Berman S. An interview with Mark Chassin. *Jt Comm J Qual Patient Saf.* 2010 Oct;36(10):475–479.

14. Jamtvedt G, et al. Audit and feedback: Effects on professional practice and health care outcomes. *Cochrane Database Syst Rev.* 2006 April 19;(2):CD000259.

15. Oujiri J, et al. Resident-initiated interventions to improve inpatient heart-failure management. *BMJ Qual Saf.* 2011 Feb;20(2):181–186.

16. Steinman MA, et al. Age and receipt of guideline-recommended medications for heart failure: A nationwide study of veterans. *J Gen Intern Med.* 2011 Oct;26(10):1152–1159.

17. Hysong SJ, Best RG, Pugh JA. Audit and feedback and clinical practice guideline adherence: Making feedback actionable. *Implement Sci.* 2006 Apr 28;1:9.

18. Dulko D. Audit and feedback as a clinical practice guideline implementation strategy: A model for acute care nurse practitioners. *Worldviews Evid Based Nurs.* 2007;4(4):200–209.

19. Trautner BW, et al. A hospital-site controlled intervention using audit and feedback to implement guidelines concerning inappropriate treatment of catheter-associated asymptomatic bacteriuria. *Implement Sci.* 2011 Apr 22;6:41.

20. Staton LJ, et al. Peer chart audits: A tool to meet Accreditation Council on Graduate Medical Education (ACGME) competency in practice-based learning and improvement. *Implement Sci.* 2007 Jul 27;2:24.

21. Accreditation Council on Graduate Medical Education. Home Page. Accessed Oct 17, 2012. http://www.acgme.org/acgmeweb/.

22. American Board of Medical Specialties. Fact Sheet: American Board of Medical Specialties (ABMS) and the ABMS Maintenance of Certification® (ABMS MOC®) Program. Accessed Oct 17, 2012. http://www.abms.org/News_and_Events/Media_Newsroom/pdf/ABMS_Fact_sheet.pdf.

23. Nolte E. *International Benchmarking of Healthcare Quality: A Review of the Literature.* Santa Monica, CA: RAND Corp., 2010. Accessed Nov 26, 2012. http://www.rand.org/pubs/technical_reports/TR738.html.

24. Chassin MR, et al. Accountability measures—Using measurement to promote quality improvement. *N Engl J Med.* 2010 Aug 12;363(7):683–688.

25. Joint Commission Center for Transforming Healthcare. Targeted Solutions Tool for Hand Hygiene. Accessed Oct 17, 2012. http://www.centerfortransforminghealthcare.org/tst_hh.aspx.

26. Cherry MG, et al. Features of educational interventions that lead to compliance with hand hygiene in healthcare professionals within a hospital care setting. A BEME systematic review: BEME Guide No. 22. *Med Teach.* 2012;34(6):e406–420.

27. Kiefe CI, et al. Identifying achievable benchmarks of care: Concepts and methodology. *Int J Qual Health Care.* 1998 Oct;10(5):443–447.

28. Weissman NW, et al. Achievable benchmarks of care: The ABC™s of benchmarking. *J Eval Clin Pract.* 1999 Aug;5(3):269–281.

29. Kiefe CI, et al. Improving quality improvement using achievable benchmarks for physician feedback: A randomized controlled trial. *JAMA.* 2001 Jun 13;285(22):2871–2879.

30. Holman WL, et al.; Alabama CABG Study Group. Alabama coronary artery bypass grafting project: Results of a statewide quality improvement initiative. *JAMA.* 2001 Jun 20;285(23):3003–3010.

31. Holman WL, et al. Alabama coronary artery bypass grafting project: Results from phase II of a statewide quality improvement initiative. *Ann Surg.* 2004 Jan;239(1):99–109.

32. Houston TK, et al. Implementing achievable benchmarks in preventive health: A controlled trial in residency education. *Acad Med.* 2006 Jul;81(7):608–616.

33. Estrada CA, et al. A web-based diabetes intervention for physician: A cluster-randomized effectiveness trial. *Int J Qual Health Care.* 2011 Dec;23(6):682–689.

34. Jarvis WR. The Lowbury Lecture: The United States approach to strategies in the battle against healthcare-associated infections, 2006: Transitioning from benchmarking to zero tolerance and clinician accountability. *J Hosp Infect.* 2007 Jun;65 Suppl 2:3–9.

35. World Health Organization. Implementation Manual: WHO Surgical Safety Checklist. World Alliance for Patient Safety. 2008. Accessed Oct 17, 2012. http://www.who.int/patientsafety/safesurgery/tools_resources/SSSL_Manual_finalJun08.pdf.

36. Messahel FM, Al-Qahtani AS. Benchmarking of World Health Organization surgical safety checklist. *Saudi Med J.* 2009 Mar;30(3):422–425.

37. CMS to measure safe surgery checklist use: Hospitals and surgery centers to report on structural measure. *The Joint Commission Perspectives on Patient Safety.* 2012 Sep;32(9):4.

38. Sexton JB, et al. The Safety Attitudes Questionnaire: Psychometric properties, benchmarking data, and emerging research. *BMC Health Serv Res.* 2006 Apr 3;6:44.

39. Webster PD, et al. Using quality improvement to accelerate highly active antiretroviral treatment coverage in South Africa. *BMJ Qual Saf.* 2012 Apr;21(4):315–324.

40. Griffin FA. 5 Million Lives Campaign. Reducing methicillin-resistant *Staphylococcus aureus* (MRSA) infections. *Jt Comm J Qual Patient Saf.* 2007 Dec;33(12):726–731.

41. Boushon B, et al. *Transforming Care at the Bedside How-to Guide: Reducing Patient Injuries from Falls.* Cambridge, MA: Institute for Healthcare Improvement, 2008. Accessed Oct 17, 2012. http://www.ihi.org/knowledge/Pages/Tools/TCABHowToGuideReducingPatientInjuriesfromFalls.aspx.

42. Schal M, et al. *How-to Guide: Improving Transitions from the Hospital to the Clinical Office Practice to Reduce Avoidable Rehospitalizations.* Cambridge, MA: Institute for Healthcare Improvement, Jun 2012. Accessed Oct 17, 2012. http://www.ihi.org/knowledge/Pages/Tools/HowtoGuideImprovingTransitionsHospitaltoOfficePracticeReduceRehospitalizations.aspx.

Chapter 6

BUILDING ON CHANGE: CONCEPTS FOR IMPROVING ANY CLINICAL PROCESS

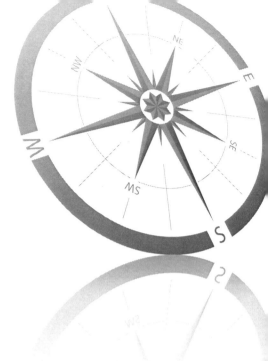

Rebecca S. Miltner, Jeremiah H. Newsom, Paul B. Batalden, Julie K. Johnson, Eugene C. Nelson, Patricia A. Patrician

Until you can see a different reality, you are hard-pressed to do anything differently.
—John Kelsch[1]

As novice practitioners achieve mature professional competence, they approach clinical pattern recognition and problem solving with increasingly reflective and integrative forms of reasoning. In a recursive and largely spontaneous process that Donald Schön refers to as "reflection-in-action,"[2] seasoned professionals combine inquiry, intervention, and evaluation to generate higher-order conceptions of complex clinical realities.[3] Whereas novice clinicians register isolated details of history and physical exams and apply formal algorithms to solve standard problems, experienced practitioners combine technical facility with intuitive appreciation and derive elegant therapeutic strategies that are both creative and clinically sound.

Earlier chapters introduced practice-based learning and improvement with a similar developmental trajectory in mind. The work of quality innovation is well supported by tools such as the Clinical Improvement Worksheet (Chapter 3) and the Clinical Value Compass (Chapter 4), but experienced practitioners of improvement will appreciate the extent to which such instruments are the means rather than the ends in the important work of enhancing health care value. With increased experience in quality improvement, clinicians' initial algorithmic view of systemwide patterns and processes grows increasingly reflective and intuitive. For example, a charge nurse who is just learning improvement methods may want to increase the number of patients who are discharged by noon. She tackles this problem with other members of the microsystem in a systematic way, using the newly learned improvement tools. However, she gets bogged down with the process of making sure they use the improvement tools correctly and in the proper sequence, which frustrates physician members of the team who see the process as wasting their time because they believe a reminder system may be all that is needed to "fix" the problem. On the other hand, an experienced clinical nurse leader who has completed many improvement projects using the same tools may approach this same problem in a more flexible manner. She has worked with the hospitalists before on other projects and recruits one of them to help colead this team. She also asks a floor nurse and unit secretary who have been valuable team members in previous work to join the team, and she delegates to them specific tasks that draw on their personal strengths. The team examines the current process first and decides on several potential changes that can be made without much effort or money, and they create a list of more complex ideas to work on if simpler ones don't work completely. The team uses easily obtainable data to monitor success and provides frequent feedback to the teams. However, the clinical nurse leader is flexible with the sequencing of these activities so that they best fit the unit work flow and take advantage of the context. For example, a particular test of change may be delayed if the unit secretary who monitors the data is on vacation that week. The nuance of balancing improvement techniques and contextual issues is gained over time and experience with improvement projects.

This chapter explores underlying change concepts that support the generation and elaboration of specific improvement ideas. A case study in which an interprofessional team works to improve mobility for hospitalized patients illustrates change-concept thinking that serves to both broaden and deepen the clinician's understanding of improvement intervention possibilities. Readers are encouraged to reflect on their own improvement experiences and to draw higher-level connections between past and future opportunities for learning and change. This chapter also examines specific principles that connect individual improvement projects to larger-scale organizational change and sets the stage for case studies of health system improvement that are explored in subsequent chapters.

Change Concepts

The ability to design and to rapidly test change is an essential capability of professional learning environments.[4-6] New design ideas—or certainly those with sufficient merit to be tested—arise from individual or collective reflection on processes now in place, with attention to high-leverage steps whose modification will enhance work quality and efficiency. Chapter 2 demonstrated how to generate multiple ideas for change from perspectives inside the system. These perspectives (for example, of clinicians, nurses, receptionists, administrators, patients, or other stakeholders) provide necessary insight into the process of care as experienced by workers themselves. But these same participants can also step back and view their work from outside the processes. Imagine an industrial assembly line or workshop, and now imagine a catwalk or viewing deck that traverses this same space. Imagine, finally, the value to participants of moving back and forth, every day, between these parallel spaces, between the workstation where processes are known experientially and the viewing deck where those same processes are understood analytically.

The opportunities for learning, making, and leading improvement are greatly enhanced by such perceptual shifts.[7]

De Bono has characterized this shifting of perspectives in greater detail and has discovered in this reframing a rich source of underlying concepts that become generators of specific improvement ideas.[8] If we understand the underlying concept on which a specific idea is based, we can use this concept to brainstorm multiple new options for action. Health professionals will recognize in this formulation a restatement of clinical reasoning processes that become increasingly natural with growing experience. Consider the example in Sidebar 6-1 (page 75) that links underlying generic concepts to specific intervention ideas. De Bono describes the value of a generic concept (X) and its relation to specific ideas (A, B, and C). This model can be conceptualized as a path forward on a main route, X, with three specific branch routes labeled A, B, and C. Similarly, a core concept labeled X might lead to many ideas labeled A, B, and C.

As Sidebar 6-1 illustrates, when we travel a road or pursue an idea, we are likely to encounter junctions of choice for new and different paths. After we have committed ourselves to a single idea, we risk narrowing our perspective to this one channel (as would have occurred in our example if Dr. Hart in the story had insisted only on increasingly aggressive pharmacologic solutions). Although such single-minded commitment is sometimes appropriate, there is often more benefit to be derived from what de Bono calls *lateral thinking*—a form of reasoning that invites us to pull back to the underlying concept, to clarify this concept by naming it, and to then imagine alternative paths forward.[8]

Change-concept thinking is well suited to the delivery and improvement of patient care. Experienced clinicians routinely apply taxonomies of diagnosis and intervention, and reflective practitioners grow increasingly facile in movements left or right (backward and forward) along these clinical branches. The case in Sidebar 6-1 offers a most elementary example. At more sophisticated levels, such thinking can and should be built into formal process-focused quality improvement initiatives.

Sidebar 6-1. Reducing Cardiovascular Risk

Dr. Hart* is reevaluating Andrew Jones, a 45-year-old office manager with untreated hypertension and elevated serum cholesterol. Mr. Jones is 30 pounds overweight and acknowledges that both his stressful job and his troubled marriage distract him from self-care. He eats "on the run," sometimes skipping meals and then overcompensating with whatever junk food is available at the workplace vending machines. At today's office visit, as during his prior visit, Mr. Jones's blood pressure is elevated to 155/90.

Dr. Hart is concerned about this blood pressure reading and about Mr. Jones's cardiovascular risk in general. She persuades Mr. Jones that his blood pressure needs to be reduced, and she invites him to brainstorm ideas that will support this goal. The "main route" along which they begin their brainstorming (route *X* in Figure 6-1 below) is "blood pressure control" (or, even farther upstream, general "cardiovascular risk reduction"). Together, they come up with several initial ideas:

A. Initiate an antihypertensive medication.
B. Begin an exercise routine at the local health club.

C. Join a work-based dietary counseling program.

Mr. Jones quickly selects option *A*, the antihypertensive medication, because he believes that this route will be simplest and most effective, with the least impact on his hectic schedule. However, at his follow-up appointment two months later, his blood pressure remains high despite compliance with the prescribed regimen, and he is experiencing unpleasant side effects from the medication.

At this point, instead of pushing farther down pathway *A* (another medication), Dr. Hart prudently "pulls back" to the underlying concept *X* and suggests an alternative path forward: *B* (exercise regimen), *C* (dietary program), or even a possible *D* (a new idea such as marital therapy or personal counseling to manage psychosocial stressors).

---

* Names of all persons are fictitious.

Figure 6-1. Change Concept–Idea Relationship

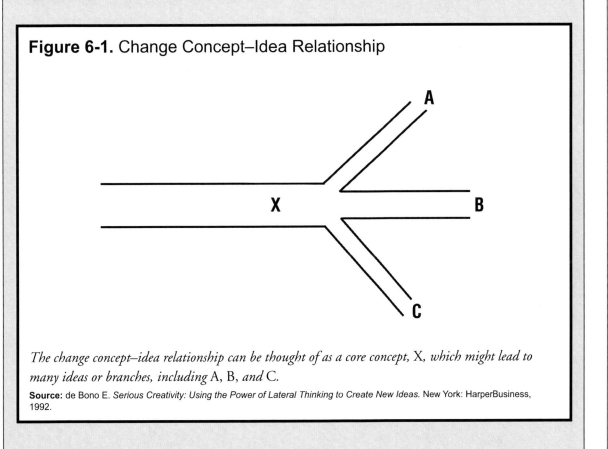

The change concept–idea relationship can be thought of as a core concept, X, *which might lead to many ideas or branches, including* A, B, *and* C.

Source: de Bono E. *Serious Creativity: Using the Power of Lateral Thinking to Create New Ideas.* New York: HarperBusiness, 1992.

Langley and colleagues have incorporated de Bono's underlying concepts into a framework that specifically supports improvement-oriented change. They have characterized these common pathways as *change concepts,* which they define as general categories or approaches to change that stimulate more specific improvement ideas.[9] A useful taxonomy of such change concepts has been developed, and Langley et al. have now identified four categories of improvement with 72 generic change concepts that can be applied to improvement design across a wide spectrum of work settings, including health care. The 72 generic change concepts have 10 general groupings that are outlined in Figure 6-2 (page 77), and each category has specific change concepts that fall under them. For example, concepts grouped around elimination of waste include, but are not limited to, eliminate things that are not used, eliminate multiple entry, recycle or reuse, and match the amount to the need. These concepts are further characterized in the case study and figures that follow.

Readers might find that the generic change concepts outlined by Langley et al. give a name to changes that have already been locally identified, or they might help clarify thinking about where in the local process new changes should be initiated. Remember, however, that change concepts cannot serve as a substitute for serious thinking about local processes of care. If practitioners have information and clear ideas about where process improvement is required, this knowledge and judgment should be trusted. Change concepts can jump-start stalled thinking or redirect it, but of course they must never supplant that thinking from the perspectives of those involved in the process to be changed.

Case Example: Using Change Concepts to Maintain Mobility of Hospitalized Patients

An interprofessional team consisting of physical therapists, hospitalists, nurses, hospital administrators, and a geriatrician came together to find ways to maintain previous mobility in hospitalized inpatients. This team's work demonstrated the utility of change-concept thinking in quality innovation and cost reduction.

In this example, core process analysis was guided by use of tools such as brainstorming and the Clinical Value Compass Worksheet[10] (described in Chapter 4), and idea generation was enriched through explicit attention to underlying change concepts. Improvement work is the responsibility of all health care workers and can be effectively implemented by individual practitioners, informal professional groups (working separately but in parallel), or well-coordinated interprofessional teams. Because of the complexity of this clinical issue, this group chose a team-based approach, but in other settings both individuals and informal groups have found the use of change concepts to be similarly fruitful.

Outcomes: Select a Population

The inpatient mobility team specified its aims with respect to achievement of clinical, functional, satisfaction, and cost outcomes that were superior to current outcomes. Low mobility (defined as bed rest and bed-to-chair activity only) is common among hospitalized patients and is associated with a host of adverse outcomes, including functional decline, increased risk of falls, increased length of stay, and a concomitant increase in community care needs upon discharge. In this facility, a study of hospitalized patients showed that in a 24-hour period, they spend an average of 83% of the day lying in bed.

The team set the goal that by hospital day 2, all patients for whom it is not contraindicated will be ambulating a minimum of 100 feet and ideally 300 feet per day. This goal applied to all patients who were ambulatory within the two weeks prior to admission.

Process: Analyze the Process

By constructing a flow diagram, the inpatient mobility team analyzed caregiving processes that produced current results. This diagram helped the team visualize specific steps in the process of ensuring that hospitalized patients ambulated daily. Figure 6-3 (page 78) illustrates this high-level flowchart. This work enabled each team member to become more fully cognizant of the complexity of this process of care. Specifically, the team realized that there was little coordination between

Figure 6-2. A Worksheet for Generating Specific Change Ideas

Change Concept Grouping	Idea for Change
1. Eliminate waste.	
2. Improve work flow.	
3. Decrease cycle times.	
4. Change the work environment.	
5. Address customer problems.	
6. Meet customer expectations.	
7. Reduce costs.	
8. Manage variation.	
9. Eliminate mistakes.	
10. Delight customers.	

Select one or two of these change concepts to help identify an area or a process for change and then design a specific change.

Source: Adapted from Langley GJ, et al. *The Improvement Guide: A Practical Approach to Enhancing Organizational Performance*, 2nd ed. San Francisco: Jossey-Bass, 2009.

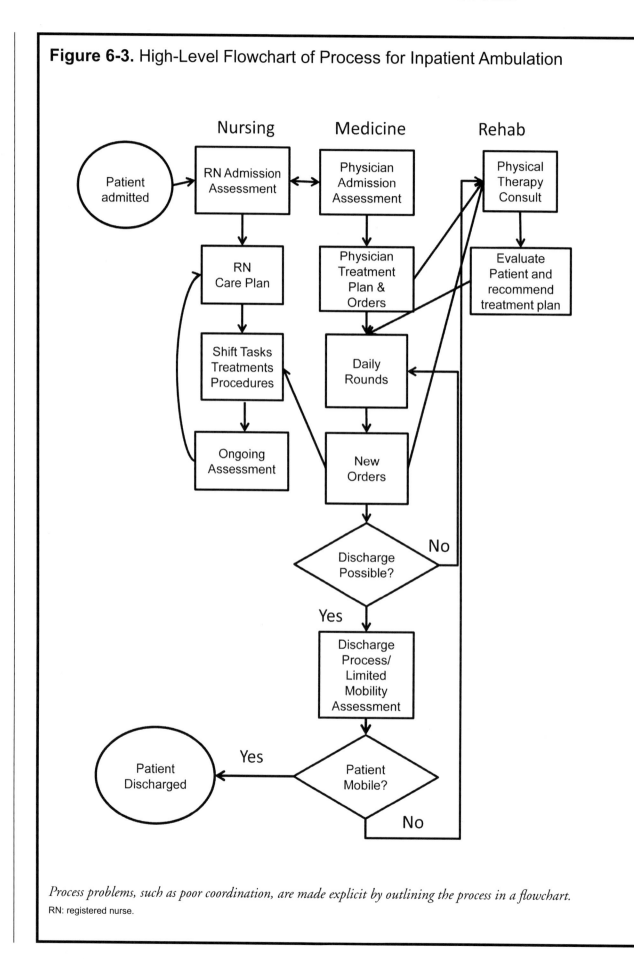

Figure 6-3. High-Level Flowchart of Process for Inpatient Ambulation

Process problems, such as poor coordination, are made explicit by outlining the process in a flowchart.

RN: registered nurse.

disciplines related to patient ambulation and little attention to the importance of ambulation in the plan of care.

Changes: Generate Change Ideas

The process of generating change ideas often occurs in parallel with the process analysis. As the inpatient mobility team discussed the work flow, several ideas emerged spontaneously for improvement of specific processes.

To optimize both efficiency and effectiveness of this critical third step on the Clinical Improvement Worksheet—"What ideas do we have for changing what is done (process) to get better results?"— the team worked with six broadly identified categories: care providers, patients/families, physical environment/equipment, leadership and finance, policies and procedures, and training and education. Over the course of several meetings, the team members silently wrote down their improvement ideas. These improvement ideas came from many sources: personal experience, professional knowledge, direct observation, literature review, and clinical benchmarking.

The team members discussed their ideas first and then grouped the ideas into underlying change concepts to further clarify their ideas for specific application to the current process. This interactive and iterative activity generated a long list of ideas and issues, creating a pool of opportunity that reinforced the feeling within the team that there was an acute need to change the current process. The team members began with specific ideas, then stepped back to identify underlying concepts, and finally used their insight from this dual perspective to generate many more specific ideas. The team leader chose this approach explicitly due to the interprofessional nature of the team to ensure that all members had the opportunity to offer ideas from their perspective. Discussion about the broader concepts after the specific idea generation allowed the team members to find common ground across disciplines. An alternative approach is to begin with generic change concepts themselves and use these concepts to directly initiate the brainstorming.

Some team members worked with the team facilitators to take the ideas and display them

on a new high-level flowchart of the ambulation process map. This flowchart enabled the entire team to visualize opportunities for greatest potential leverage, where specific pilot tests of change might yield the greatest impact on outcomes and costs.

Figures 6-4 and 6-5 (pages 80 and 81) illustrate the product of this last exercise and offer a particularly practical formulation for design of change in clinical processes. All of the previously listed generic change concepts are identified and correlated with specific sites of potential change in the ambulation process of care. These same general change concepts have been used by individual practitioners and by formal improvement teams to stimulate efficient redesign and improvement in multiple patient care settings.

When the mobility team reviewed its work, several important but unanticipated benefits had been achieved, including the following:

- A "savings account" of great ideas had been built up, permitting individual team members (or smaller pairings of individuals, or the entire team) to pursue successive small tests of change over time using the Plan–Do–Study–Act (PDSA) methodology—PDSA cycle 1, PDSA cycle 2, and so on.
- Deeper appreciation of the current process had been linked with specific ideas for both improvement of discrete elements within that process (incremental first-order change) and redesign of the entire process (innovation, or second-order change).
- The powerful generic change concepts had been explored in detail and could now be applied more routinely and thoroughly, not only in maintaining inpatient mobility but also in the management of other important processes.
- Empowered by these general insights and specific ideas, the team proceeded to Step 4 on the Clinical Improvement Worksheet: selecting a first test of change.

Pilot: Select a Change for Pilot Testing

To select its first pilot test, participants reviewed the specific change ideas listed earlier in Figure 6-4 and then asked, "Where is the leverage for

Figure 6-4. Sample Worksheet of Change Concepts for Improving Inpatient Ambulation

Underlying Generic Change Concepts	Idea for Change
1. Eliminate waste.	*Have assistive devices such as walkers readily available on nursing unit instead of requesting from rehabilitation services.*
2. Improve work flow.	*Build ambulation order sets into admission order sets to include distance and frequency.*
3. Decrease cycle times.	*Consult physical therapy early in hospitalization if patient has mobility risks.*
4. Change the work environment.	*Develop a competency-based training program for nursing and physical therapy staff about improving inpatient mobility.*
5. Address customer problems.	*Use motivational interviewing techniques to encourage ambulation.*
6. Meet customer expectations.	*Include patient in daily plan of care and write ambulation goals on whiteboard in patient room.*
7. Reduce costs.	*Schedule mobility appointments during times of decreased unit activity to optimize availability of staff without additional resources.*
8. Manage variation.	*Standardize policies and procedures to include role clarification among nurses, nursing assistants, and physical therapists.*
9. Eliminate mistakes.	*Prohibit "bed rest" orders in computerized provider order entry without mandatory justification.*
10. Delight customers.	*Increase resources for mobility awareness, including marketing to patients, families, and staff.*

This worksheet is a filled-in example of the one shown in Figure 6-2.

Source: Adapted from Langley GJ, et al. *The Improvement Guide: A Practical Approach to Enhancing Organizational Performance,* 2nd ed. San Francisco: Jossey-Bass, 2009.

Figure 6-5. Change Concepts Applied to Inpatient Ambulation

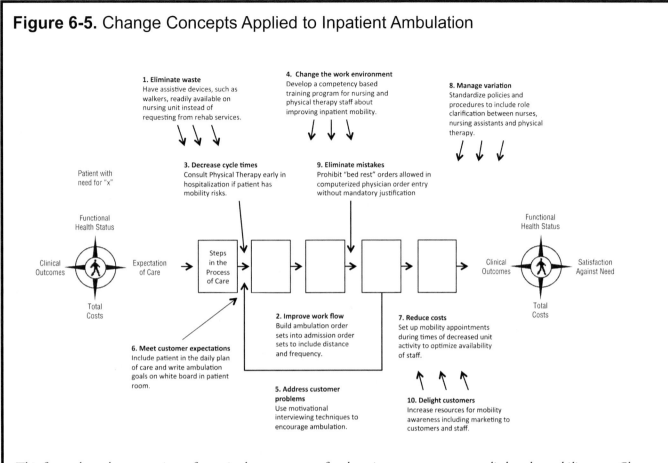

This figure shows how groupings of generic change concepts for changing any process are applied to the mobility case. Change concepts, specific improvement ideas for changing the inputs, action steps, outcomes, and the entire process are superimposed on the core clinical process represented as a flowchart of ambulation of inpatients. The blank boxes represent generic steps in the entire process; the team working on a particular setting would have mapped out the entire process in more detail.

change? What changes will have the largest effect on patient safety? on current resource use? on current reliability? on other subprocesses (including influence or ripple effects on the entire collection of interlinked subprocesses)?" Next, team members considered the relative complexity of pilot alternatives (illustrated in a "ramp of complexity" that has been described by Langley et al.[11]), and they addressed the critical question: "What is the largest feasible change that we can test, that we predict will lead to improvement, and that we can implement by a near certain date?"

In light of these several considerations, the team decided that the first test of change would combine two specific ideas for change: physician order for specific ambulation distance and frequency and inclusion of the patient in the plan of care

development and implementation. The team considered this two-part test a doable first step in the change process that would have the largest effect on patient safety, required little additional resource use, and had potential to build process reliability, as this microsystem was staffed by six hospitalists who supported this team's work.

The remaining improvement ideas were held for further exploration and potential use in subsequent cycles of change.

Change in Organizations

The inpatient mobility case example is presented as if in a vacuum, with only minimal discussion of the greater health care organization in which the improvement team functioned. But real-world improvement work does not occur in a vacuum.

Health care organizations are complex systems, and practitioners of improvement must understand how change occurs within this context. How do local changes affect the larger organizational system, and how does that system "push back"? Organizational change is difficult because it usually requires coordinated actions among many individuals and departments in the midst of other competing organizational requirements. It is important to understand organizational change not only for successful implementation of change but also for maintenance over time and for successful adaptation in new settings.[12]

Resistance to Change: A Marker of Identity?

Internal resistance to change is common, and most of us can recount experiences when even obvious tension for change was insufficient to motivate key players within a system. What is the source of this internal resistance?

Both individuals and organizations are keenly sensitive to challenges to their own identity and recognize that perceived perturbations to the integrity of this identity—the introduction of material that is "strange" or "foreign"—might naturally trigger a self-protective response. This identity-preserving action is common to all living organisms and systems and is well illustrated in the familiar antigen–antibody response. When presented with an antigenic challenge, our bodies typically recognize the offending agent as foreign, and our immune cells generate specific antibodies to neutralize the threat. Although the defensive function of this antibody response is apparent to all who study cellular systems, the same response also serves as a biologic expression of self-identity. In the very act of preserving its own boundary between self and other, the organism defines this boundary more precisely.

In similar fashion, when individuals and organizations express resistance to change, they could well be communicating a need to preserve the integrity of boundaries against potentially threatening, and certainly "foreign," ideas or interventions. The resistance itself might initially frustrate champions of change and innovation, but as in the case of molecular antibodies, this defense also sends a potentially valuable signal of self-identity. Skilled leaders of change, when sensitive to such signals, can use them to better explore the system itself, and this exploration might in turn support change strategies that can be embraced by all participants. The message for practitioners of clinical improvement is, therefore, that when resistance is encountered, it should not be resisted in turn. Rather, it should be examined, understood, and actively engaged.

Readiness for Change

Readiness for change has been described in several ways, including at the individual and organizational levels. Lewin's classic change management model proposes a three-stage model of unfreeze, change, refreeze.[13] In the first stage, unfreezing of current mind-sets occurs through creating a motivation to change. Such motivation can be facilitated in many ways, including increasing dissatisfaction with the status quo, creating a sense of urgency to change, or taking advantage of a crisis situation. In health care, this readiness to change may be the consequence of a series of adverse patient events. But no matter the catalyst, creating this readiness for change is essential to successful change efforts.

In the second stage, the discomfort from the first stage allows opening of possibilities for change. To manage this stage successfully, it is important that people understand how change will benefit them personally. This phase requires active intervention and encouragement from change leaders to assist other members of the group to see the benefits of change.

Finally, in the last stage, most people have come to accept the change, but the structures to support the change have to be made permanent. Policies and procedures as well as physical and organizational infrastructure need to be aligned to support the change so it becomes part of the culture of the organization. Lewin's change model is important for health care professionals who are working to improve care, but the simplicity of the model may not be sufficient within the complex health care environment. Another model may offer some additional insight to professionals working to improve care.

A Model for Change

Readiness for change can be viewed from the individual, group, or organizational level. Building on work from several disciplines, Weiner proposes a theory for organizational readiness for change that addresses both the organization members' commitment to change (change commitment) and the collective belief that there is the capability to do so (change efficacy).[14] Weiner's model of organizational readiness for change is shown in Figure 6-6 below. Weiner suggests that organizational readiness for change is a function of how organizational members value the change and three characteristics of implementation: task demands, resource availability, and the current situation. The value that organizational members assign to the change can be based on a sense of urgency, personal benefit, customer benefit, and/or formal or informal leadership support.

To assess this belief that the proposed change can be implemented, Weiner suggests asking the following three questions[14]:

1. Do we know what it will take to implement this change effectively?
2. Do we have the resources to implement this change effectively?
3. Can we implement this change in the current situation?

This theory indicates that the concept of organizational readiness for change is situational.

Team members may be ready and able to implement some change ideas but not prepared to implement others. Preparing for change requires assessment of three areas: the organization members' value of the change, their belief that they can implement the change, and the contextual factors that support the implementation of change.

The team described in the previous case study experienced this balance between the organization members' commitment to change and the belief that resources were available to support the change. Several team members had individually championed efforts to improve inpatient mobility in a number of ways, including improving physical therapy availability, conducting research about inpatient mobility, and championing the use of safe patient handling equipment. Such individual efforts did not bring about real and sustained change. However, the improvement team came together following a class on developing aims for improvement in which inpatient mobility was used as an example. Discussion after the class led to pulling together all the interested parties into a process action team. In addition, the organization had recently hired a new director of quality resources who championed new clinical improvement teams. Growing financial constraints within the organization provided further impetus for the change. Improving mobility for hospitalized patients could reduce length of stay as

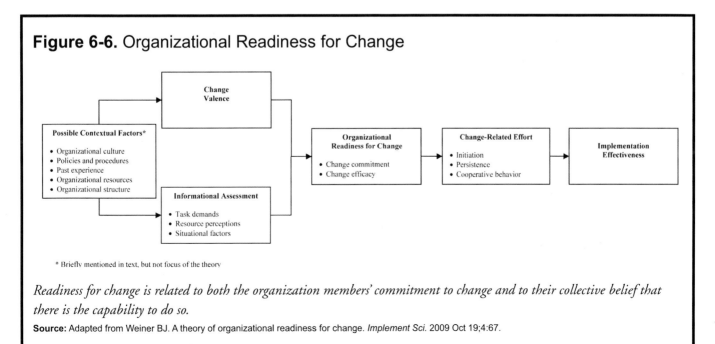

Figure 6-6. Organizational Readiness for Change

Readiness for change is related to both the organization members' commitment to change and to their collective belief that there is the capability to do so.

Source: Adapted from Weiner BJ. A theory of organizational readiness for change. *Implement Sci.* 2009 Oct 19;4:67.

well as postdischarge needs, such as home physical therapy.

The "stars aligned" in this organization to bring several disciplines together to work on a long-term project to improve mobility for hospitalized patients. Change is not always successful in the first attempt, but taking advantage of the opportunities that arise within an organization can improve the odds of success.

Creating Change

John P. Kotter has studied changes that failed. By exploring the underlying causes of such failures, Kotter identifies essential leadership qualities that support an organization's achievement of meaningful change. His important work *Leading Change*[12] describes eight stages in the process of improvement leadership. The reader will recognize in Kotter's eight-stage model several similarities to the clinical improvement strategy we have promoted in earlier chapters of this book. His model includes the following phases:

1. Establish a sense of urgency.
2. Create a guiding coalition.
3. Develop a vision and strategy.
4. Communicate the change vision.
5. Empower broad-based action.
6. Generate short-term wins.
7. Consolidate gains and produce more change.
8. Anchor new approaches in the culture.

The tools we have presented throughout this book can support practitioners' improvement work in each of Kotter's eight stages. Further explication of these ideas appears in Chapter 7.

Building on Change

In a world that itself is continually changing, the survival of health care systems depends on their capacity to initiate and manage internal change. Clinicians not only must anticipate but also should embrace and strive to lead such inevitable transitions, whether they occur in direct patient care, in professional development, or in continuous improvement of health care delivery systems.

This chapter has explored higher-order manifestations of change as they appear in health care settings. It has introduced both generic change concepts (that underlie specific improvement ideas) and models of organizational readiness for change.

Chapter 7 explores the maintenance of such change in increasingly complex systems of care. It explores how to sustain our gains and how to extend them. Chapter 8 links these clinical and system changes to the developmental transitions of practitioners themselves and the learning of teamwork that is so germane to changing clinical processes. It asks what processes and structures support clinicians' growing competence as agents and leaders of change. These are not simple questions, nor are there simple, one-size-fits-all answers. But the well-being of our patients and the need to improve the quality and safety of our health care delivery systems require earnest exploration and intelligent action.

References

1. Personal communication between the author [P.B.B.] and John Kelsch, Chief Quality Officer, Xerox Corporation, Stamford, CT, 1992.
2. Schön DA. *The Reflective Practitioner: How Professionals Think in Action.* New York: Basic Books, 1983.
3. Taylor BJ. *Reflective Practice for Healthcare Professionals: A Practical Guide,* 3rd ed. Berkshire, England: Open University Press, 2010.
4. Argyris C, Schön DA. *Organizational Learning II: Theory, Method, and Practice.* Reading, MA: Addison-Wesley, 1996.
5. Kolb DA, Rubin IM, Osland J. *Organizational Behavior: An Experiential Approach.* Englewood Cliffs, NJ: Prentice Hall, 1991.
6. Marquardt MJ. *Building the Learning Organization: Achieving Strategic Advantage Through a Commitment to Learning,* 3rd ed. Boston: Nicholas Brealy, 2011.
7. Parks SD. *Leadership Can Be Taught: A Bold Approach for a Complex World.* Boston: Harvard Business School Press, 2005.
8. de Bono E. *Serious Creativity: Using the Power of Lateral Thinking to Create New Ideas.* New York: HarperBusiness, 1992.
9. Langley GJ, et al. *The Improvement Guide: A Practical Approach to Enhancing Organizational Performance,* 2nd ed. San Francisco: Jossey-Bass, 2009.
10. Nelson EC, et al. Improving health care, Part 1: The Clinical Value Compass. *Jt Comm J Qual Improv.* 1996 Apr;22(4):243–258.
11. Langley GJ, Nolan KM, Nolan TW. The foundation of improvement. *Quality Progress.* 1994 Jun;27(6):81–86.
12. Kotter JP. *Leading Change.* Boston: Harvard Business School Press, 1996.
13. Lewin K. *Field Theory in Social Science: Selected Theoretical Papers.* New York: Harper, 1951.
14. Weiner BJ. A theory of organizational readiness for change. *Implement Sci.* 2009 Oct19;4:67.

Chapter 7

IMPLEMENTING, SPREADING, AND SUSTAINING ORGANIZATIONAL CHANGE

Patricia A. Patrician, Grant T. Savage, Rebecca S. Miltner, Velinda Block, Robert Weech-Maldonado

If you do what you've always done, you'll get what you've always gotten.
                                                            —Tony Robbins[1]
No man ever steps in the same river twice, for it's not the same river and he's not the same man.
                                                            —Heraclitus[2]

Organizational improvement cannot happen without change. From small tests of change within a single microsystem to sweeping changes in governmental reimbursement policy that serve as an external motivator for organizational transformation, change is an inevitable part of our work in health care. It will not serve us well to attempt to maintain the status quo, which may mean maintaining suboptimal structures and processes. However, sometimes innovation simply fails.[3] The failure of innovation implementation in health care may lie not in the manner in which the changes were implemented but in the lack of attention to the spread and sustainment of change throughout organizations and systems.

To improve health care safety and quality, leaders must be well versed in the application of change principles to the practice setting. Change must be facilitated, monitored, and actively managed to "take hold" in an organization. This chapter builds on the change ideas and change concepts introduced in Chapters 2 and 6 as well as tools and techniques to use in quality improvement, such as the Clinical Improvement Worksheet and Clinical Value Compass (Chapters 3 and 4, respectively) and benchmarking (Chapter 5). This chapter reviews the theoretical basis and pragmatic strategies for implementing, spreading, and sustaining change that lead to health

care improvement. The Institute for Healthcare Improvement (IHI) Framework for Spread will be discussed. Two examples highlighting innovation spread and sustainment will be presented. Knowledge about change processes and pitfalls will better equip quality improvement leaders to actualize their safety and quality innovations and to maintain quality over time.

Why Is Change So Difficult?

In the previous chapter, we discussed the organization's readiness for change. But there is also a need to pay attention to the individual's readiness for change. There are many reasons individuals resist change, including discomfort, inadequate resources or planning, lack of incentives, and a leadership void.

Discomfort

Change is uncomfortable; there is a certain amount of anxiety associated with the unknown, particularly when individuals' sense of power, status, or employment security is threatened. Thus, there is a strong emotional basis for maintaining stability and status quo. Indeed, Saint et al. point out the "active resisters" and "organizational constipators" who impede improvement efforts.[4] Kotter discusses the "if it ain't broke, don't fix it" mentality that dominated businesses in the mid-twentieth century.[5] Globalization, technology, and a faster pace of life made ideas about change and improvement more inevitable, but not necessarily easier. Resistance to change, covered in more detail in Chapter 6, should be expected and embraced.

Inadequate Planning

Repenning and Sterman use the term *improvement paradox* to explain why, no matter how effective the intended improvements, implementation fails.[6] They explain that quality improvement programs cannot be purchased as premade, ready-to-use solutions; rather, they must be developed from within the organization.[6]

Usually, organizations devote insufficient resources to implementing, spreading, and sustaining change and add the related responsibilities to employees' existing workloads. This is what makes improvement work so difficult—and nearly impossible if added on as an extra responsibility for a handful of workers in the absence of a plan for implementation.

Repenning and Sterman suggest a balance between the pressure to speed up work processes and the time spent on finding ways to improve production processes.[6] A tension arises from this attempt to create a balance, similar to the tension that arises from taking time to plan versus jumping right into action. Improvement can happen only when people and resources are specifically freed up from their usual tasks to work on improvement. In other words, the team must build in time for improvement, not just work harder or longer. Process improvement is like preventive maintenance, which in the short term is time-consuming and may be expensive but in the long term greatly reduces costs. Similarly, positive changes that result from process improvement may save time and money in the long run.

Lack of Incentives

When individuals perceive that a change does not benefit them directly, they are more likely to resist efforts to change. *Change agents,* or *champions,* are people from within the organization who serve as leaders, or catalysts, for change.[7] These change champions must understand what would motivate their colleagues to change their practices or behaviors. Sometimes motivation is encouraged for organizations through payment reimbursement initiatives, whereby organizations are penalized for unfavorable outcomes, such as cuts in Medicare reimbursement for hospital-acquired complications. From the individual provider perspective, however, it may not be the economic benefits of the change so much as the improvement of patient care quality and improvement of work processes that motivates change efforts.

Heath and Heath describe several ways to rally individual support for a change idea: evoke emotion; focus on outcomes; paint a clear, concrete, realistic picture of the goal; and create short-term wins.[8] One effective way to evoke emotion is to tell stories or show videos that describe why the current reality is not working.[9] For example, in the wake of a serious adverse event, a full review of the event may include inviting the patient and family members to the organization to tell their perspective about what happened and what the event meant to them.[10] It is more difficult to resist the changes that need to occur when the current processes result in devastation to others. Emotionally laden testaments such as these can be useful if tailored specifically to the change one wants to bring about. Providing graphically arrayed data on outcomes can also powerfully convey the need for improvement, particularly when combined with benchmarks from other organizations (*see* Chapter 5). Individuals will be more likely to adopt changes if they not only understand but can visualize the goal of the change and if they can actually see the progress over time.

Leadership Void

Change for the sake of improvement is made more difficult in organizations that lack transformational leaders. As Kotter noted, paralysis occurs when an organization has too many managers and not enough leaders because management's job is to maintain the status quo and minimize risks, whereas the goal of leadership is to envision a future beyond the status quo and take the necessary risky steps to create new systems, to innovate.[5] Change is difficult in a system in which leadership is lacking, but having the wrong type of leadership at the helm is equally challenging. Nembhard and associates examined leadership as a component of innovation implementation failure in health care and explained why the traditional boss–employee relationship (that is, transactional leadership) is not well suited for change implementation.[3] This approach uses a reward-versus-punishment mentality to motivate employees to do their respective jobs and is more aligned with the definition of *management* than *leadership*.

Transformational leadership, however, uses consensus building among followers as a motivational strategy. According to Kouzes and Posner, transformational leadership has the following key attributes: challenging the status quo, inspiring others to create a shared vision, empowering others to act on the vision, modeling the way, and providing meaningful rewards. This leadership style shifts organization members' focus from their individual goals to such collective goals as innovation implementation.[11] Such leaders not only inspire their followers but also understand the resources required to implement change and provide the requisite support.

In describing why change is so difficult, we begin to see what it takes to implement change effectively in an organization. The next section reviews Kotter's framework for implementing change, along with practical strategies to ensure success.

Implementing Change

Noted retired Harvard Business School professor John P. Kotter developed a linear model of change implementation on the basis of his research on change in more than 100 companies.[5] He noted that successful change and improvement required sequential steps. His eight-step model, summarized in Sidebar 7-1 (above right), has been applied successfully in health care organizations.[12,13]

Establish a Sense of Urgency

The first step, establishing a sense of urgency, is critical to creating the momentum needed for change. Kotter states that 50% of companies fail in this step.[5] He offers practical tips to create urgency by

---

> ## Sidebar 7-1. Kotter's Eight Stages of Change
>
> John P. Kotter's linear model of change implementation includes the following eight steps:
> 1. Establish a sense of urgency.
> 2. Create a guiding coalition.
> 3. Develop vision and strategy.
> 4. Communicate the change vision.
> 5. Empower broad-based action.
> 6. Generate short-term wins.
> 7. Consolidate gains and produce more change.
> 8. Anchor new approaches in the culture.
>
> **Source:** Adapted from Kotter JP. Leading change: Why transformation efforts fail. *Harvard Business Review*, 1995 Mar–Apr;73(2):61.

setting high benchmarks, displaying data that show poor performance relative to that of competitors, allowing financial losses, eliminating company excesses, and insisting that managers and others talk regularly to unhappy customers. The successful outcome of this step is catching the attention of the organization's leaders and workforce to pave the way or increase the level of readiness for change.

Create a Guiding Coalition

The next step in the change process is to create a guiding coalition. Successful change does not happen simply because the leader says so. Organizational change can be actualized only through team efforts. Therefore, team members need to be carefully selected to be representative of the individuals who will implement the change and others who will be affected by it. The change coalition should include people who hold positional power as well as informal power, content experts among the professional groups involved, leaders and managers, and patients if appropriate. It is ideal to create this coalition from individuals who can work as a team; those with large egos or those who tend to "stir the pot" need not join the team! After the right people are identified, the team will need time and direction to build trust and develop a common goal through joint meetings and other activities.

Develop Vision and Strategy

Developing a vision for the new future that will result from the change and a strategy to get there is the next step in the change process. Vision statements take some time to develop and should not be attempted in one meeting—usually multiple meetings will be necessary. There are many ways to get started with developing a vision, and perhaps common to most methods is brainstorming and getting the entire team to participate in what the future should look like as a result of the change. An effective vision is one that is imaginable, desirable, feasible, focused, flexible, and communicable. It should be short and memorable. Strategies then can be developed from the vision, with concrete steps that outline how to attain the vision and the time line to reach it.

Communicate the Change Vision

Communicating the change vision seems rather mundane but is critical to do—and to do often. Ineffective organizational communication relies on passive dissemination via e-mail, memos, or newsletters and assumes that people need to be told only once about the change vision. We all are acutely aware that e-mail takes up a significant portion of our workday and that often messages are deleted without being read. We also know that posted notices often are ignored. Providers and other health care team members need to hear a simple, consistent message from the leaders in the organization and the change team members in multiple venues for it to resonate and be heard. Those who work shifts may need brief huddles at shift change to obtain important messages. Text messaging and websites may be beneficial tools for getting the message across. A variety of methods will be necessary. To get staff nurses' attention, nurse managers have been known to post important information in the staff lounge and even the restroom! The vision must be communicated through both words and actions because there is nothing more powerful than leading by example.

Empower Broad-Based Action

Empowering broad-based action refers to removing the barriers that hamper workers when attempting to initiate a change. Often organizational structures such as the authority, resource allocation, information, and personnel systems need to be realigned to accommodate the change. Workers may need additional training to institute the change if new knowledge, skills, or attitudes are required.[14] Finally, if any supervisors are found to be undermining change efforts and disempowering staff members, this behavior must be confronted and corrected immediately.

Generate Short-Term Wins

Because seeing the fruits of one's labor is a powerful motivator, the next step in the change process is generating short-term wins. Short-term wins, which should be built into the strategy for accomplishing the change vision, serve several purposes. These wins provide the evidence to health care providers that the sacrifice is well worth it, and the wins undermine critics. Analyzing the short-term gains helps fine-tune strategies as well as reward the change agents and team, keep supervisors on board, and build momentum by turning the naysayers into believers of the cause. The final two steps in Kotter's change model—consolidating gains and producing more change, and anchoring new approaches into the culture—are more appropriately discussed in the sections that follow under "Spreading Change" and "Sustaining Change," respectively.

Spreading Change

After change has been initiated and is successful in one area, how can we actively spread it to other areas in the same organization?

Consolidate Gains and Produce More Change

Kotter provides a partial answer in the seventh step of his model, consolidating gains and producing more change. If the change appears to be working, this success motivates others to become involved with the process and often results in more help with the change. The involvement of others also helps with streamlining new processes as the innovation takes hold within the organization.

Rogers studied how innovations diffuse throughout society and devised a five-stage process of how this occurs.[7] First, practitioners need knowledge about what changes need to be implemented and how these changes have worked in other settings. To obtain such knowledge, practitioners must understand their own system and what processes and outcomes are falling short of the goals, and they must examine research and other evidence to determine the possibilities for change. Second, practitioners need to persuade other individuals that a change is needed. This second stage is similar to Kotter's first step of establishing a sense of urgency about the change, and it is heavily influenced by change agents within the system. Rogers's third stage involves a decision to adopt the change. The fourth stage is change implementation. The fifth stage is confirmation that the change is indeed having its desired effect.

One of Rogers's unique contributions to this literature is his characterization of innovation adopters. With regard to change, he suggests that individuals fall into several strata and that the population distribution of these strata follows a bell-shaped curve[7]:

• Innovators
• Early adopters
• Early majority
• Late majority
• Laggards

Innovators make up a small proportion of the population (that is, on the right tail of the bell curve) and are described as visionaries who see potential for change and actively seek out new information.[15] *Early adopters* are those who seek out new information and enjoy testing new ideas in their practice. They are also opinion leaders with informal power that allows them to influence their coworkers. It is imperative for change leaders to engage the innovators and early adopters in the beginning stages of planning for change, as it is these individuals who in turn will sway others to join the improvement effort. The *early majority* is the critical mass of individuals (that is, in the central portion of the bell curve) who can be rather easily swayed by the early adopters. The *late majority* are skeptics who are averse to risk and change. This group needs additional attention from management to become convinced that the value of the change makes it worth implementing, and they will do so only if they are rather sure the change is

working. Finally, the *laggards* are the minority of individuals (that is, on the left tail of the bell curve) who have the greatest difficulty with change. They will need extra persuasion or, if they remain unable or unwilling to change, may need to be removed from the organization. Knowing how to address the characteristics of the various types of adopters can assist managers and leaders with spreading improvement.

The IHI Framework for Spread, illustrated in Figure 7-1 (page 90), has been used successfully in many improvement projects and offers perhaps the most comprehensive model for spreading change in health care organizations.[16] This framework is formulated from Rogers's diffusion of innovations work and draws upon social learning, self-change, and social marketing theories. The Framework for Spread posits that individuals within a clinical microsystem must take the lead in innovation implementation and that the leader's job is to help them envision the change, help them see the need for change, and support them in attaining and spreading the change.

In the Framework for Spread, leadership is essential for spreading improvement throughout the organization. In a hospital, for example, leadership should include the executive team as well as the *executive sponsor*—the individual who has the ultimate responsibility for day-to-day management and execution of spreading the innovation. The leadership team sets the vision for spreading the change, realigns organizational priorities given the change, and empowers the executive sponsor to act. Middle managers have key roles in supporting the change, including removing barriers to change and assisting their employees in implementing the change.

Key components to consider are the change ideas and setup for the spread. Any change consists of "better ideas" that not only need to be articulated clearly but also need to be carefully supported. The case must be made for why the change is necessary and that evidence exists to show how these better ideas are, in fact, better than the status quo. *Setup* refers to understanding the context in which the spread will take effect. The microsystems within which the change will be implemented and

Figure 7-1. Framework for Spread

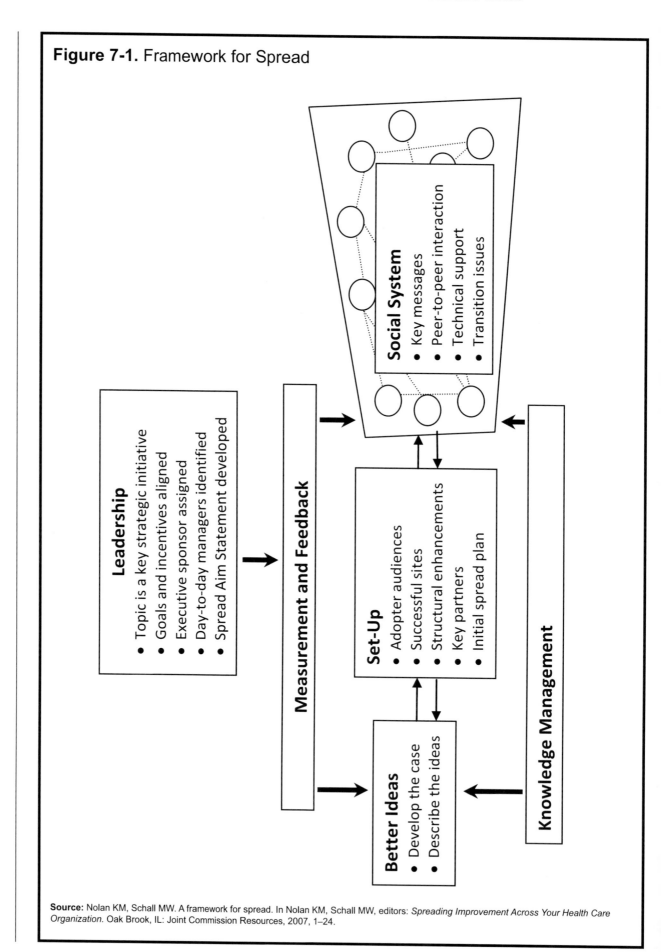

Source: Nolan KM, Schall MW. A framework for spread. In Nolan KM, Schall MW, editors: *Spreading Improvement Across Your Health Care Organization.* Oak Brook, IL: Joint Commission Resources, 2007, 1–24.

spread need to be understood from the perspective of the health care providers, other personnel, patients, and the processes through which they are interconnected. A thorough assessment of the setup will enhance the strengths of the change initiative and highlight those areas of weakness that need to be addressed, such as additional resource requirements. When both these components are in place, the stage will be set for a favorable environment in which change will spread.

Another aspect of the Framework for Spread is the social system, which influences how the change initiative will be communicated within the health care organization, including technology support and the messaging or marketing of the change. This component emphasizes the role of innovators and early adopters in serving as change champions and rallying others to action. Measurement, feedback, and knowledge management are essential to the successful spread of change. Measurement of the change progress is important because it indicates whether the change is making a difference and meeting the intended aim or if any unintended consequences arise. Feedback based on measurement should go to all levels of personnel and is important in sustaining interest in and passion for the change. Moreover, as new knowledge becomes available regarding the spread of the change, this knowledge should be shared with the staff. Chapter 5 expands on an approach for measurement and feedback to compare practices and benchmarking to communicate results, identify best practices (early successes from innovators), and create tension for change.

Sustaining Change

All the work that has gone into implementing and spreading the change will be for naught if the change does not last. Therefore, let us now turn our attention to the final key component of a successful organizational change: sustaining the change.

Anchor New Approaches in the Culture

According to Kotter, anchoring new approaches in the organization's culture is the final step in the change process because the reshaping of

norms and values comes at the end of the change process.[5] Institutionalizing change embeds the new process in the organization through linkages with job descriptions, performance appraisals, quality improvement structures and processes, and patient care documentation templates. For example, making quality and patient safety a core competency for all employees within the organization, with clearly defined performance criteria for each job type, can facilitate embedding the change in the organization. For a housekeeper, core competencies might include ensuring that hand hygiene dispensers are always functional and full on the assigned unit; for a nurse, they might include being held accountable for hourly rounding for patient safety. New approaches become part of a culture only after they have proven to work better than the old way and after they become part of day-to-day business processes. Thus, it is critical to alter system processes, such as evaluation and promotion, to align with the change; otherwise, people will fall back into their previous behavior patterns, and the old culture will reassert itself. Making it easy for personnel to adopt the change, while making it difficult for personnel to revert back to the prechange processes, will help sustain the change. In the Framework for Spread, this is called a "forcing function."[17] Engaging health care providers and other key personnel, who are usually the most knowledgeable about how best to integrate the change into daily processes, is essential.

This stage of change requires ongoing communication and support from leadership. Focus groups and surveys to get feedback from health care providers, other personnel, and patients are beneficial. Continued monitoring of processes and outcomes of the change is equally important.

Case Studies from the Field

We have reviewed how changes occur in organizations, how they take hold, and how they are spread and sustained. We conclude the chapter with two case studies from the field—the first on implementing a change, and the second on sustaining a change within a large academic medical center.

Case Study: Implementing Change
Addressing Improvements in Patient Experiences

According to the Institute of Medicine, high-quality health care should be safe, effective, patient-centered, timely, efficient, and equitable.[18] Patient-centeredness includes assessing the patient experience and satisfaction to ensure that health care organizations are meeting patient expectations and their health care needs. An important tool to assess the patient experience with inpatient care is the Hospital Consumer Assessment of Healthcare Providers and Systems (HCAHPS). Sponsored by the Agency for Healthcare Research and Quality (AHRQ) and the US Centers for Medicare & Medicaid Services (CMS), HCAHPS is a standardized survey that asks a random sample of recently discharged patients about important aspects of their hospital experience. HCAHPS includes six composite measures (communication with physicians, communication with nurses, staff responsiveness, pain control, communication about medications, and discharge information), two individual report items (cleanliness of hospital environment and quietness of hospital environment), and two global items (recommendation of hospital to friends and family and overall rating of hospital).[19]

Hospitals are increasingly focusing on improving the patient experience as shown by their HCAHPS scores. CMS currently includes HCAHPS scores as one of the publicly reported measures in Hospital Compare, a website that allows patients to compare hospitals based on their quality.[20] Furthermore, HCAHPS has been incorporated into the Hospital Value-Based Purchasing (VBP) program (beginning in the 2013 fiscal year) as part of the Patient Protection and Affordable Care Act of 2010. Under the VBP initiative, hospitals will receive incentive payments based on their performance on HCAHPS scores and improvement in those scores.[21] Patient-centered hospitals are expected to use HCAHPS scores in conjunction with other quantitative and qualitative data to enhance their patient experience.

We describe here the efforts of an academic medical center to improve the patient experience. The hospital is located in a major metropolitan area of the Midwest in the United States and serves an ethnically diverse patient population. Recent public reporting of HCAHPS data shows the hospital performing worse than its competitors, particularly with respect to nurse communication and discharge information. Some evidence suggests that the relatively poor performance is beginning to affect the hospital's market share. This concern has prompted the chief executive officer (CEO) and the executive team to meet with department heads to discuss a systemwide strategy to address the HCAHPS performance. The meeting group decides to appoint a Patient Experience Improvement Task Force to lead the organizational effort; its members would act as change champions throughout the system. The task force would be led by the vice president for quality improvement and would include representatives of various clinical and functional departments as well as management and staff. The CEO calls a town hall meeting to discuss the hospital's HCAHPS performance and introduce the task force as an organizational effort to improve the patient experience. The CEO's vision is that the hospital becomes the premier health care organization and the hospital of choice in the market.

As a first step, the task force examines the HCAHPS data by unit and patient demographics. Data show wide variations in patient experiences across departments, with members of racial or ethnic minority groups reporting worse experiences with care. Subsequently, separate focus groups are conducted with patients, nurses and other staff, and physicians to understand the root causes of the problem. Patients express frustration with the "lack of caring and empathy" and what they perceive as negative attitudes. They also complain that they leave the hospital without sufficient information on care after discharge. Some minority patients also stress language barriers and the limited and often poor quality of interpreter services. On the other hand, nurses and staff complain of being overburdened with multiple demands and pressures, administrative paperwork, equipment failures, staffing and supply shortages, and often inadequate training.[22] As a result, nurses feel overloaded and emotionally drained. It is clear to the task force that substantive changes are necessary if the hospital is to improve the patient experience, and toward this end it decides to embark on a multipronged strategy to address both patient and staff concerns.

The hospital launches a "JUST ASK" campaign, in which patients are encouraged to ask questions relating to their care, ranging from availability of various food selections to medication management. Nurses and staff are trained and encouraged to do the following[23]:

- Establish rapport
- Make proper introductions
- Reinforce the hospital's commitment to meeting patients' needs
- Set proper expectations and address any temporary setbacks to the extent possible
- Communicate reasons for delays in any procedures

To improve its discharge communication process, the hospital implements the following strategies:

- Develop a patient checklist to ensure comprehensive communication at discharge
- Review patient handouts to ensure that they are written at appropriate health literacy levels
- Enhance website content to include frequently asked questions upon hospital discharge
- Institute postdischarge follow-up calls to ensure that patients have no immediate concerns or queries

Departments are asked to establish HCAHPS goals and an action plan to address those goals. Staff members are empowered to implement changes, and it is made clear to them that their suggestions and input are highly valued. Furthermore, constant interaction between department leaders and direct care workers is stressed. Additional personnel are provided to departments that are struggling with staff shortages, making it clear that the hospital is prepared to make substantial initial investments to improve patient experiences with care. Recruitment of a diverse workforce is made an organizational priority, and nurses and staff are trained on cultural sensitivity and the hospital's language access policy.

The task force evaluates HCAHPS scores by

department on a monthly basis to monitor changes and identify areas for improvement. Six months after the task force is instituted, it meets with the CEO and presents an interim report. This report is discussed in another town hall meeting, where units showing the best performance and greatest improvement in HCAHPS scores are recognized. Acting on one of the task force's recommendations, the hospital decides to appoint a patient advocate, whose responsibility includes addressing patient complaints and helping administrators and staff improve quality and patient satisfaction. To ensure that patient-centered care remains an organizational priority, it is incorporated into job descriptions, performance evaluations, and incentive systems.[22] The hospital strives for continuous improvement in patient experiences through its quality improvement processes.

Case Study: Sustaining Change
A Shared Governance Transformation

Shared Governance (SG) is a decision-making model that has been used in health care organizations since the early 1980s as a means to empower staff and engage them in the decision-making process.[24] Authority and power are shared mutually with those who have a vested interest in the outcome of the decision. SG is not participatory management but rather an accountability-based process that gives practitioners the authority to address issues that directly relate to their practice. With the creation and implementation of SG models, hospitals found that patient care outcomes improved and staff nurses were more highly satisfied with their roles. For hospitals that seek designation as a Magnet facility by the American Nurses Credentialing Center, it is essential that they have a strong SG model in place to demonstrate structural empowerment as well as transformational leadership.[25] As part of its journey to Magnet designation, the University of Alabama at Birmingham (UAB) University Hospital, a large academic medical center in Birmingham, Alabama, needed to implement an SG structure that would demonstrate the empowerment of its staff. The Professional Nurse Practice Council (PNPC) was developed in 2003 and brought together staff nurses from around the organization. Through their monthly meetings and work teams, they focused on three main areas: creating a positive healthy work environment, efficiency in care, and professional practice. Although the group members were fully engaged, they were not truly empowered. The PNPC was used as a sounding board or a place to gather input, but little if any decision making occurred within the council.

When a new chief nursing officer joined the organization in 2007, she was concerned about both the function and the outcomes of the PNPC and saw that most decisions were still being made by the nursing leaders, including decisions that affected clinical practice. Such practice was contrary to the function and purpose of the council and did not empower staff nurses to act to improve care. After spending six months observing and assessing the organization, she identified the need to develop a new Nursing Vision statement to create the foundation for change and align priorities. A Vision Team was created, which included staff from all levels of the organization. Under the leadership of the chief nursing officer, the team members developed a Vision draft, which they took out to hundreds of nurses for input through focus groups. This process ensured a strong level of ownership of the Vision by many individuals in the organization rather than sole ownership by the chief nursing officer. After the Vision was complete, the team identified development of a true Shared Governance model as a critical first goal.

To effectively develop a new SG model that engaged frontline nursing staff, a work team was formed. The team members were charged with reviewing the literature and models across the country and developing a proposed model that would focus on clinical nursing practice at both the global and unit levels. During this process, the team discovered that some organizations were successfully using a congressional model and determined that this model would be ideal for their own organization. They called the new model Nursing Practice Congress (NPC) because it was built on the concept of having all specialties represented in the decision-making process for clinical nursing issues.

The group would be chaired by a staff nurse leader who was allocated 20 hours a week to effectively run the NPC. The framework of the NPC focused on true empowerment as nursing practice issues and changes were all funneled to the congress. The NPC representatives were taught how to use evidence-based practice and multidisciplinary teams to drive their decisions.

In its first two years of existence, the NPC reviewed 36 concerns and formed work groups around 29 specific practice issues.[25] These work groups developed 19 specific clinical practice changes, which were successfully implemented hospitalwide.[25] One example of these practice changes included moving from disposable to reusable blood pressure cuffs in appropriate patient populations. This change not only reduced costs but also contributed to the hospital's "green" initiatives by reducing hospital waste. Another example focused on patients who had difficult IV access. Through the work of the NPC, an algorithm was developed to guide the nurse in terms of alternatives when escalation was needed. The organization is now working to implement a Nursing Practice Congress for each of the hospital's 55 nursing units and is expected to have that work accomplished by the end of 2013.[25]

The success and sustainability of this SG journey is tied directly to Kotter's change model. Through the creation of a shared Vision for nursing and the engaging of staff from all levels to serve as a guiding coalition, nurses could begin to see their opportunity for true empowerment. The NPC was able to have quick early wins that demonstrated to all that the process for making decisions had changed in this organization.

References

1. ThinkExist. Anthony Robbins Quotes. Robbins T. Accessed Oct 18, 2012. http://thinkexist.com/quotation/if_you_do_what_you-ve_always_done-you-ll_get_what/222354.html.

2. ThinkExist. Heraclitus of Ephesus Quotes. Heraclitus. Accessed Oct 18, 2012. http://thinkexist.com/quotation/no_man_ever_steps_in_the_same_river_twice-for_it/208269.html.

3. Nembhard IM, et al. Why does the quality of health care continue to lag? Insights from management research. *Academy of Management Perspectives.* 2009 Feb;23(1):24–42.

4. Saint S, et al. How active resisters and organizational constipators affect health care–acquired infection prevention efforts. *Jt Comm J Qual Patient Saf.* 2009 May;35(5):239–246.

5. Kotter JP. *Leading Change.* Boston: Harvard Business School Press, 1996.

6. Repenning NP, Sterman JD. Nobody ever gets credit for fixing problems that never happened: Creating and sustaining process improvement. *California Management Review.* 2001;43(4):64–88.

7. Rogers EM. *Diffusion of Innovations,* 5th ed. New York: Free Press, 2003.

8. Heath C, Heath D. *Switch: How to Change Things When Change Is Hard.* New York: Broadway Books, 2010.

9. Lobos AT, et al. An implementation strategy for a multicenter pediatric rapid response system in Ontario. *Jt Comm J Qual Patient Saf.* 2010 Jun;36(6):271–280.

10. Schwappach DL. Engaging patients as vigilant partners in safety: A systematic review. *Med Care Res Rev.* 2010 Apr;67(2):119–148.

11. Kouzes JM, Posner BZ. *The Leadership Challenge,* 3rd ed. San Francisco: Jossey-Bass, 2002.

12. Hendrich A, et al. The Ascension Health journey to zero: Lessons learned and leadership perspectives. *Jt Comm J Qual Patient Saf.* 2007 Dec;33(12):739–749.

13. Britto MT, et al. Combining evidence and diffusion of innovation theory to enhance influenza immunization. *Jt Comm J Qual Patient Saf.* 2006 Aug;32(8):426–432.

14. Schilling L, et al. Kaiser Permanente's performance improvement system, Part 1: From benchmarking to executing on strategic priorities. *Jt Comm J Qual Patient Saf.* 2010 Nov;36(11):484–498.

15. Gibbons W, et al. Eliminating facility-acquired pressure ulcers at Ascension Health. *Jt Comm J Qual Patient Saf.* 2006 Sep;32(9):488–496.

16. Nolan KM, Schall MW. A framework for spread. In Nolan KM, Schall MW, editors: *Spreading Improvement Across Your Health Care Organization.* Oak Brook, IL: Joint Commission Resources, 2007, 1–24.

17. Render ML, et al. Evidence-based practice to reduce central line infections. In Schilling L, editor: *Implementing and Sustaining Improvement in Health Care.* Oak Brook, IL: Joint Commission Resources, 2009, 49–55.

18. Committee on Quality of Health Care in America, Institute of Medicine. *Crossing the Quality Chasm: A New Health System for the 21st Century.* Washington, DC: National Academy Press, 2001.

19. US Centers for Medicare & Medicaid Services. HCAHPS: Hospital Care Quality Information from the Consumer Perspective. (Updated: Jun 15, 2012.) Accessed Oct 18, 2012. http://www.hcahpsonline.org/home.aspx.

20. US Department of Health & Human Services. Hospital Compare. (Updated: Oct 11, 2012.) Accessed Oct 18, 2012. http://www.hospitalcompare.hhs.gov.

21. US Centers for Medicare & Medicaid Services. *HCAHPS Executive Insight.* Accessed Oct 18, 2012. http://www.hcahpsonline.org/Executive_Insight/.

22. Barr JK, et al. Using public reports of patient satisfaction for hospital quality improvement. *Health Serv Res.* 2006 Jun;41(3 Pt 1):663–682.

23. Planetree; Picker Institute. Patient-Centered Care Improvement Guide. Accessed Oct 18, 2012. http://www.patient-centeredcare.org/inside/abouttheguide.html.

24. Porter-O'Grady T. *Implementing Shared Governance: Creating a Professional Organization.* St. Louis: Mosby-Year Book, 1992.

25. American Nurses Credentialing Center (ANCC). *Application Manual: Magnet Recognition Program®.* Silver Spring, MD: ANCC, 2008.

Chapter 8

HEALTH PROFESSIONALS ENGAGED IN PRACTICE-BASED LEARNING AND IMPROVEMENT

**Maryjoan D. Ladden, Deborah Gardner, Connie Lopez,
Michael A. Tijerina, Benjamin B. Taylor, Carlos A. Estrada**

*The time is right. . . . Our resources are limited, and it's our obligation to determine and apply
our health resources as effectively and robustly as possible in ways that produce better care outcomes
for patients. As the health care community is looking for new strategies, and new ways of organizing
to optimize our efforts—teamwork is fundamental to the conversation.*

　　　—Mary Wakefield, PhD, RN, Administrator, Health Resources and Services Administration

*The health care system will not be able to keep pace with these explosive changes unless it moves to a team-based
care model. . . . But the delivery system cannot make that shift effectively until the education system begins to
train new health professionals in collaborative practice.*

　　　—George Thibault, MD, President, Josiah Macy Jr. Foundation

Practice-based learning and improvement (PBLI) is the reflective and iterative integration of observation and action, during clinical care, to enhance the knowledge and high-quality delivery of that care in every encounter (as described in Chapters 1 and 2). A fundamental aspect of PBLI is the ability to continually improve quality and safety within the constraints and resources of clinical settings. Hence, PBLI and continuous quality improvement (CQI) are best viewed from a perspective of all involved in the care of the patient. PBLI-CQI is the work of everyone and is often done in teams.

In this chapter we provide an overview of the importance of teamwork and collaboration for both organizational leaders and health care workers. We also review effective components of teamwork and strategies to increase collaboration as well as interprofessional education and its core competencies. Finally, we provide examples from a large integrated health care delivery system on programs for team training and training techniques and resources.

Sidebar 8-1 on pages 98–99 illustrates a practical and successful approach of health professionals engaged in PBLI. Hospitals and other acute care facilities are examples of complex organizations. Hospital units care for the sickest patients. Physicians, nurses, respiratory therapists, pharmacists, social workers, and other health care professionals usually staff each unit. Regardless of hospital size, location, private or public organizational status, university affiliation, or any other characteristic, each hospital unit aims to provide the best possible care within available resources.

Teamwork and Collaboration

The Institute of Medicine and other national organizations have highlighted the critical importance of collaboration, teamwork, and interprofessional education to improve patient quality and safety; however, the progress for wider implementation has been slow.

Health care professionals must apply a skill set not routinely emphasized in medical education: teamwork

Sidebar 8-1. Case Study: Teamwork and Collaboration at a Large Academic Medical Center

The Setting

The University of Alabama at Birmingham (UAB) University Hospital, a 900-bed tertiary care facility in a large metropolitan area, provides primary and specialty care for adults. Each hospital unit provides care for a defined patient population. Hospital units include critical care units (surgical, medical, cardiac, neurological), medicine units (general, hematology/oncology, pulmonary), and others.

Medical care is provided in covered services with physicians in training (residents and fellows), students, and a small group of hospitalists. Nurses work in a defined unit, and each unit has a nurse manager and a medical director.

The Challenges

University Hospital is a large, complex academic medical center with more than 40 inpatient care units. As compared to national benchmarks from University Health Consortium (UHC), standard measures of quality of care were lower than similar academic medical centers. The quality metrics did not reflect the dedication, commitment, and expertise of the medical and nursing staff as well as other health professionals. The mandated reporting of quality metrics was emotionally difficult to accept and hard to understand.

Physicians, nurses, and pharmacists were busy working on multiple projects. However, each unit created its own set of local priorities and addressed the emergent issues, resulting in a large variability of patient care.

The Solution

In January 2010, hospital units started forming unit-based clinical leadership teams. The main charge was to define and focus on the most important quality issues at each unit level. Each unit-based team included the medical director, nurse manager, nurse educator, and pharmacist.

Each unit's quality dashboard was based on the UHC quality and accountability scorecard (safety, mortality, effectiveness, patient-centered). Initially, the hospital created a set of basic quality metrics that spanned all hospital unit settings. Each unit then started out with a basic set of goals, priorities, and metrics. The quality dashboard enabled team members to own and understand their respective units. Each unit-based team was expected to understand the way that care is delivered in their own units, rather than all the metrics and other care processes in other units.

The first project focused on patient safety. The main aim was to eliminate hospital-associated infections—specifically, central line–associated bloodstream infections and catheter-associated urinary tract infections—in intensive care units and on medical and surgical floors. Such infections among hospitalized patients increase mortality. Evidence was available on best strategies to decrease infections. The project was catalyzed by the public reporting mandate by the US Centers for Medicare & Medicaid Services (CMS);* institutions are to publicly report health care–acquired conditions, and payments for such conditions would not be allowed by the federal government effective July 1, 2011.

Progress to Date

As of March 2012, most units had formed unit-based clinical leadership teams. Although not formally

continued on next page

and collaboration. In daily practice, physicians, nurses, and other professionals must work together to care for patients. When health care professionals understand and respect one another's roles, they are better able to communicate and work together—and ultimately to provide better care.[1,2]

A *team* is defined as two or more individuals who have specific roles, perform interdependent tasks, are adaptable, and share a common goal. *Interprofessional education* is defined as occasions when two or more professions learn with, from, and about each other to improve collaboration.[3] Interprofessional education, teamwork, and collaboration in clinical practice have been

associated with improved patient and staff satisfaction, improved recognition and treatment of clinical disorders, improved patient safety, and reduction in clinical errors.[2,4–6]

In a recent report of national stakeholders including government, nonprofit organizations, and a wide range of health care professional organizations, factors that would foster teamwork and collaboration were found to include the following[1]:

- Emphasis on quality of care and patient safety
- Focus on the patient. Patients expect their health care team to work together.
- Promise of health care reform. In addition to

Sidebar 8-1. Case Study: Teamwork and Collaboration at a Large Academic Medical Center, *continued*

measured, culture change is apparent; medical directors and nurse managers continually discuss and review opportunities, and team members have taken more ownership in the process. At the quality and safety hospital meetings—led by the chief quality officer—early successes from unit-based teams were identified, best practices were summarized and disseminated, and standardized approaches across units were implemented. For example, urinary catheter management was standardized across all units; the total number of days patients have an indwelling urinary catheter (Foley) continues to decrease, as illustrated in Table 8-1 (below).

Lessons Learned

- An organized approach to improve quality, safety, and patient satisfaction at the unit level aligned institutional priorities with a focused activity.
- A healthy competitive nature drove improvement. The unit-specific quality dashboards provided a transparent comparison of quality components and created accountability.
- Communication of success stories and best practices by leadership further recognized teams and increased engagement. Communication to the board of directors also ensured further support.

Table 8-1. Total Number of Days with Indwelling Urinary Catheter (Foley)

Unit	Jan 2012	Feb 2012	Difference	% Change
A	474	387	87	−18.4
B	813	737	76	−9.3
C	642	540	102	−15.9
D	192	195	3	+1.6
E	179	123	56	−31.3
F	144	108	36	−25.0
G	606	555	51	−8.4
H	124	82	42	−33.9
I	88	86	2	−2.3
J	59	59	0	0.0
Total	**3,321**	**2,872**	**449**	**−14.0**

the Patient Protection and Affordable Care Act (2010), which provided incentives for care coordination, improved transitions of care, and focus on preventive care, private insurers also provide incentives for teamwork care.

- Aging population with more complex and chronic medical problems
- Evolving scientific knowledge

However, in the same report, barriers identified include absence of role models to work as part of a team with the relevant skill set, inadequate reimbursement and support for team-based care and interprofessional education, resistance to change as health professionals with limited experience work in teams, and logistical barriers for interprofessional education.

True interprofessional collaboration involves a negotiated agreement between health professionals that demonstrates value for the expertise and contributions that various disciplines bring to patient care. Because the majority of health professionals receive their training in teamwork and collaboration on the job rather than in a formal academic setting, it is critically important to understand how effective these practice-based interventions are in improving true interprofessional collaboration and teamwork in practice.

Components and behaviors of effective teamwork include team leadership, mutual performance monitoring, backup behavior, adaptability, team orientation, a shared mental model, mutual trust and respect, and closed-loop communication.[4,5] These components are described in Table 8-2 on page 101.[7]

High-functioning teams recognize, learn, and apply components of effective teamwork. The routine implementation of these components results in increased situational awareness. *Situational awareness* and *self-awareness* refer to a person's perception and understanding of his or her environment.

Finally, strong commitment to the organization, interest in producing the highest-quality outcomes, willingness to work collaboratively, and fostering positive personal interactions are also considered essential components for effective collaboration and increased professional satisfaction. Health care systems can design educational strategies and embed effective components into their daily work.[4]

Interprofessional Education

Interprofessional education is the process in which various disciplines learn and work with, about, and from one another to achieve the goal of collaborating to provide optimal patient care. Interprofessional education can be provided during the education of health care professionals, as graduate training, or as continuing education.

Effective interprofessional education encourages disciplines to invite collaboration and colearning while respecting the particular education, training, skills, and values of each discipline. Interprofessional education is not intended to create one skill set for multiple disciplines but to help providers understand and respect their differences and utilize these different skills most effectively in patient care.[8]

An Institute of Medicine report recommended that schools of medicine, nursing, and allied health graduate practitioners with the competencies of cooperation, collaboration, communication, and teamwork to provide care that is continuous and reliable.[9]

To promote interprofessional education and learning experiences, the following six national associations formed the Interprofessional Education Collaborative (IPEC) group: the American Association of Colleges of Nursing, Association of American Medical Colleges, American Association of Colleges of Pharmacy, American Dental Education Association, American Association of Colleges of Osteopathic Medicine, and Association of Schools of Public Health.

As shown in Table 8-3 on page 102, the IPEC panel identified four core competency domains for interprofessional collaborative practice: interprofessional communication, teams and teamwork, roles and responsibilities, and values and ethics. For comparison, the table also shows core competencies for graduate medical education (post-MD training), adult-gerontology primary care nurse practitioner, and pharmacy.

How Do Health Professionals Really Learn About Teamwork and Collaboration?

Although teamwork, collaboration, and quality and safety are formally included in the graduate competencies for medicine, nursing, and pharmacy, how well prepared are physicians, nurses, and pharmacists to work together to improve quality and safety after they complete their formal education? The answer to that question is variable.

Interprofessional learning experiences during the formative education years range from a onetime "getting to know you" experience to the more intensive—and more effective—shared classes and clinical training. Although the number of schools embracing interprofessional education has grown, the majority of schools still do not provide the depth of shared learning needed to prepare health professionals to work in a team when they get into practice. Similarly, although quality and safety have been required competencies for many years, most health professional learners have not been actively engaged in these activities while in school.[10]

Although many advocates for interprofessional education argue that it prepares health professionals in their formative education years to work together collaboratively as part of a team, the evidence linking interprofessional education to more effective

Table 8-2. Effective Teamwork Components

Component	Tasks	Example
Team leadership	Direct and coordinate activities, assess team performance, assign tasks, motivate members, facilitate team problem solving, provide performance expectations, clarify member roles, prepare for meetings, perform feedback, assist in conflict resolution.	A physician leader of the team for preventing hypoglycemia in hospitalized patients plans for the next meeting by requesting information systems to provide an updated scorecard.
Mutual performance monitoring	Develop common understanding, monitor teammate performance, identify positive behavior and mistakes, provide positive and corrective feedback.	A pharmacist from the patient-centered medical home team recognizes a problem in following results of hemoglobin testing and contacts the nurse responsible for laboratory testing follow-up.
Backup behavior	Anticipate and respond to one another's needs based on responsibilities, recognize delays, shift workload.	The nurse manager notices a surge in deliveries and shifts responsibilities of unit nurses.
Adaptability	Adjust course of action based on new information and changing conditions, recognize change in conditions, identify opportunities, scan environment, develop plans.	An intensive care unit pharmacist notices that anticoagulation management has become erratic after new infusion pumps were deployed. Pharmacists huddle with nurses to review administration protocols.
Team orientation	Prioritize team goals above individual ones, consider alternative solutions, share information, set goals as a group.	An outpatient team notices that patients scheduled for screening colonoscopy are being delayed. By sharing information, the group identifies that the new clerk was not properly trained on referrals.
Shared mental model	Know the structure and relationships between the task and members, anticipate and predict members' needs, identify changes in team or tasks, know team's goals.	At each meeting, enough time is included in the agenda to allow team members to get to know one another and what is important to them.
Mutual trust and respect	Believe all members will perform their roles and respect one another, share information, accept feedback, admit mistakes, listen to one another, speak up, keep positive attitude.	One week after a patient is seen in the teaching continuity clinic, the resident comments to the attending: "I forgot to follow up on the glucose testing on Mrs. Y last week. It is 380 mg/dL. What should I do now?"
Closed-loop communication	Confirm that information is received, follow up to ensure message received, acknowledge message received, clarify message.	A resident asks a medical student to insert a nasogastric tube in a patient. The student responds, "OK, I will insert an NG tube in Mr. X in room Y. Is that correct?"

Source: Adapted from Baker DP, et al. The role of teamwork in the professional education of physicians: Current status and assessment recommendations. *Jt Comm J Qual Patient Saf.* 2005 Apr;31(4):185–202.

Table 8-3. Core Competencies

Core Competencies for Interprofessional Collaborative Practice*	Graduate Medical Education Core Competencies†	Adult-Gerontology Primary Care Nurse Practitioner Competencies‡	Pharmacy§
• Interprofessional communication	• Interpersonal and communication skills	• The nurse practitioner–patient relationship • The teaching–coaching function	• Communication and education
• Teams and teamwork • Roles and responsibilities	• Systems-based practice	• Managing and negotiating health care delivery system	• Collaboration with patients, caregivers, and other health care professionals
• Values/ethics	• Professionalism	• Professional role	
	• Patient care • Medical knowledge	• Management of patient health/illness status • Culturally sensitive care	• Clinical problem solving, judgment, and decision making • Medical information evaluation and management • Therapeutic knowledge
	• Practice-based learning and improvement	• Monitoring and ensuring the quality of health care practice	• Management of patient populations

* Interprofessional Education Collaborative. Core Competencies for Interprofessional Collaborative Practice: Report of an Expert Panel. May 2011. Accessed Oct 18, 2012. https://members.aamc.org/eweb/upload/Core%20Competencies%20for%20Interprofessional%20Collaborative%20Practice_Revised.pdf.

† Accreditation Council for Graduate Medical Education (ACGME). ACGME General Competency Requirements. Feb 6, 2002. [Link no longer active] http://www.acgme.org/acWebsite/irc/irc_competencies.pdf. The ACGME is responsible for the accreditation of post-MD medical training programs within the United States.

‡ American Association of Colleges of Nursing. Adult-Gerontology Primary Care Nurse Practitioner Competencies. Mar 2010. Accessed Oct 18, 2012. http://www.nonpf.com/associations/10789/files/Adult-GeroPCComps2010.pdf.

§ American College of Clinical Pharmacy, Burke JM, et al. Clinical pharmacist competencies. *Pharmacotherapy.* 2008 Jun;28(6):806–815.

collaboration and teamwork in practice is not conclusive.

Few studies have evaluated the effectiveness of team training programs and other practice-based interventions on patient outcomes. A review of interventions to improve team training in hospitals found mixed results.[1] For example, in the United Kingdom, simulation-based team training in an obstetric setting found significant reductions in brachial palsy injury and reduction in time from diagnosis of uterine prolapse to infant delivery. However, another study evaluating the use of teamwork training in an obstetric setting found no reduction in the rate of adverse outcomes. The authors speculate that the differences in the length of training and emphasis in practice may explain the lack of consistent results.[1]

A systematic review noted significant differences in methods and outcome measures in the studies.[11]

Also, although positive changes in the knowledge, attitudes, and skills necessary for collaboration were reported, behavioral changes related to group interactions, problem solving, or communication skills were inconsistent.

In a more stringent Cochrane systematic review,[5] four of six studies found that interprofessional education improved working culture and patient satisfaction and decreased errors in the emergency department, improved care to domestic violence victims, and improved the knowledge and skills of clinicians caring for mental health patients. However, the studies did not demonstrate effects on other areas. Two of the studies found that interprofessional education had little to no effect on changing health professionals' behavior in practice. The authors recommended more rigorous evaluation of interprofessional education, including larger sample sizes and more appropriate control groups.[5]

Because effective interprofessional education is not the norm, it often falls to health care organizations and practice sites to retrain new health professionals in collaboration, teamwork, and quality improvement using practice-based interventions. Using the lessons learned from high-risk industries that train for hazardous situations has the potential to improve communication skills, collaborative teamwork, patient safety, and clinical outcomes. Many health care organizations have modified Crew Resource Management training, simulation, and other airline training techniques for staff development.

Research on the effectiveness of practice-based interventions to improve collaboration and teamwork is complicated by several factors. First, many terms, such as *collaboration, communication, coordination,* and *teamwork,* are used interchangeably but really have different meanings. In addition, because health care is delivered in multiple settings and contexts with different configurations of teams, defining optimal team-based care and how to measure it is challenging.

The evidence suggests that although practice-based interprofessional collaboration interventions can improve collaboration and teamwork and thus health care processes and outcomes, there are too few studies and the evidence from them is inconclusive to promote widespread adoption of one particular technique. More research

is needed to, first, identify the most effective interprofessional education methods to prepare new health professionals to work collaboratively in teams; second, develop better metrics to examine the effectiveness of practice-based interventions in actually changing health professionals' behavior in practice; and third, examine the impact of interprofessional education and practice-based interventions on improving patient outcomes.

In another review on interprofessional collaboration including physicians, nurses, and a range of health professionals, five studies were included.[12] Three studies found improvements in patient care correlated to drug use (no increase in drugs and decreased use of antidepressants and hypnotics), decreases in length of hospital stay, and decreased hospital costs. The fourth study showed no impact, and the fifth study had mixed results. In this review, the most effective interprofessional collaboration practice-based interventions were interprofessional rounds, meetings, and audits.[12]

Finally, emerging evidence suggests that team training improves clinical outcomes in combat situations, nosocomial infections, and perinatal morbidity[13]; team training also increases the quantity and quality of presurgical procedure briefings.[14] As a matter of fact, experts suggest 12 best practices for evaluation of team training that could be implemented across health care settings[15] (*see* Sidebar 8-2, below).

Sidebar 8-2. Twelve Best Practices for Team Training Evaluation

Planning
1. Start backward and use framework for evaluation in reverse (return on investment, outcomes, behaviors, learning, reactions).
2. Strive for strong experimental design.
3. When designing plans and metrics, ask the experts (frontline staff).
4. Leverage existing data.
5. Consider multiple aspects of performance.
6. Design for variance.
7. Consider organizational, team, or other factors that may help (or hinder) the effects of training.

Implementation
8. Engage players early (physician, nursing, executive leadership).
9. Plan for evaluation continuity (employee turnover).
10. Ensure that the evaluation process and trained knowledge, skills, and attitudes are valued by the organization.

Follow-up
11. Coach. Provide results to frontline providers, facilitate improvement through coaching.
12. Report results in a meaningful way.

Source: Adapted from Weaver SJ, Salas E, King HB. Twelve best practices for team training evaluation in health care. *Jt Comm J Qual Patient Saf.* 2011 Aug;37(8):341–349.

The Kaiser Permanente Experience with Quality Improvement and Team Training

Kaiser Permanente has been using team training and simulation training since 2003 to support its goal of developing an expert team from the teams of experts. Kaiser is recognized as one of the leading health care providers and not-for-profit health plans in the United States, serving approximately nine million members in nine states and the District of Columbia.

Simulation, as a teaching method, began after a team of risk and quality leaders reviewed claims data and identified five high-risk clinical areas needing improvement. Simulation allows health professionals and caregivers to practice medical procedures, critical thinking processes, and communication skills under realistic critical event circumstances without risk to actual patients. Research supports simulation-based education as an effective teaching methodology that improves learning, retention, critical thinking, and situational awareness over what would have been achieved through lecture-based teaching.

The first standardized national patient safety program at Kaiser focused on perinatal issues. Key elements of this program included a memorandum of understanding outlining the role of leadership, development of regional and local patient safety committees, collection of benchmark data using a safety attitudes questionnaire, communication training using Situation–Background–Assessment–Recommendation (SBAR) techniques, and fetal monitoring and team training using simulation. In addition, each hospital conducted emergency drills quarterly to improve and maintain collaborative teamwork and communication skills. Since the inception of this program in 2003 a significant decrease in birth-related claims has been observed.

Although simulation began as a grassroots movement, Kaiser Permanente now has several robust national simulation programs. Table 8-4 on page 105 describes such programs. According to Kaiser, the most effective programs contain the following:
- Interprofessional team training
- Standardized curriculum easily modified for various learners, needs, and environments
- Immersive and interactive training methodologies
- Tools for assessment, implementation, measuring, and sustaining the program
- A focus on cultural and performance change and not just training

Kaiser uses risk and quality data to target areas for improvement. New simulation programs follow a standardized template and are linked to clinical outcomes. Each program includes tools such as quizzes, survey evaluations, and checklists for improving team and individual skills. To ensure transfer of learning and behavioral change in the clinical setting, checklists focused on human factors or crisis resource management are also used during real emergent events.

The first program described in Table 8-4, Collaborating for Outcomes, was developed in collaboration with the Advisory Board Company. This is a multiyear culture and performance change program that requires significant leadership and staff buy-in. The other programs described were developed to improve teamwork and safety in surgical procedures and train staff or faculty instructors around critical events and perinatal issues such as shoulder dystocia and vacuum delivery. *See* Appendix F for supplementary information that goes along with each of the programs listed in Table 8-4; the information includes tools, course agendas, checklists, and evaluation surveys.

Quality Improvement and Team Training Techniques and Resources

In addition to simulation training, many organizations have instituted interdisciplinary or interprofessional rounds to provide a regular forum to improve communication and shared understanding. Interdisciplinary rounds have been associated with lower mortality rates among intensive care unit patients. Recent studies found that structured interdisciplinary rounds increased team member ratings of the quality of collaboration and teamwork climate and reduced adverse events.[2]

The use of surgical safety checklists and "daily goals" worksheets in interdisciplinary rounds has

Table 8-4. Programs Used by Kaiser Permanente to Enhance Quality and Team-Based Care

Program Name and Description	Benefits	Challenges
Collaborating for Outcomes* A multiyear culture and performance change management program designed to improve relationship dynamics and performance outcomes (service, quality, safety). The program supports health care teams on their journey to collegial partnerships.	Codesigned with staff for staff. Curriculum easily modified to meet individualized group needs. Offers diagnostic and skill-building tools, training programs, surveys and metrics, and communication strategies.	Fee for the initial train-the-trainer course facilitated by the Advisory Board Company (http://www.advisory.com). Success of program is dependent on facilitator/project management. Lacks interfacilitator rater tools for follow-up courses.
Highly Reliable Surgical Team (HRST) Program Developed in response to an unacceptable number of patients subjected to preventable harm. Grounded in human factors to encourage collaboration and consensus from each member of the perioperative team based on briefings (a short one- to two-minute pause in which members of the surgical team discuss the background of the case, assess threats and risks, and offer any other relevant information).	No cost for participants. Standardized curriculum. Evidence-based and proven to work (based on unpublished Kaiser Permanente results).	Three-day program. May require simulation equipment. Needs intensive organizational resources.
National Critical Events Team Training— Simulation Instructor (Level I) Course A three-day facilitator-training course that teaches others how to conduct Critical Events Team Training (CETT). CETT is an interprofessional training program to teach teamwork and communication skills. Elements of the program include the following: • Human factors and systems design • High-reliability organizations and teams • Simulations/debriefing	No cost for participants. Standardized curriculum. Integration of the top simulation instructor programs in the nation.	Three-day program. May require simulation equipment. Success of program is facilitator and facility dependent. Lacks interfacilitator rater tools.
National Simulation-Based Education and Training—Simulation Instructor (Level II) Course Level II aims to create instructors who use teamwork and communication training to change their hospital's/departments' culture and train others. Based on the concepts that simulation is just one methodology and is more than the manikins. This course places greater emphasis on advanced debriefing skills, instructional design, organizational alignment, measuring success, and return on investment.	No cost for participants. Standardized curriculum. Integration of the top simulation instructor programs in the nation.	Three-day program. May require simulation equipment. Success is facilitator and faculty dependent.
National Perinatal Patient Safety Programs Blended learning programs designed for learning transfer. The goal is to save lives by making expert teams.	No cost for participants. Standardized curriculum. Four-hour program.	May require simulation equipment. Success of program is facilitator and facility dependent.

* Developed by Kaiser Permanente National Patient Care Services in collaboration with the Advisory Board Company. Other programs were developed by Kaiser Permanente National Risk Management, Jeff Convissar, MD, director, and Connie Lopez, national leader. Contact the latter at connie.m.lopez@kp.org for more information. See Appendix F for supplementary information that goes along with each of the programs listed in this table; the information includes tools, course agendas, checklists, and evaluation surveys.

been found to further facilitate teamwork and improve patient outcomes. Surgical checklists provide structure to communications, thereby ensuring a shared understanding of the operative plan. Use of checklists has been shown to result in a significant reduction in inpatient complications and mortality. In addition, consistent use of daily goals worksheets during interdisciplinary rounds in the intensive care unit has demonstrated significant improvements in physician–nurse ratings of their understanding of the goals of care.[16–20]

For example, the World Alliance for Patient Safety at the World Health Organization compiled and disseminated a publicly available manual to implement the Surgical Safety Checklist.[21] The checklist identifies three phases of a surgical intervention: before anesthesia induction ("Sign In"), before skin incision ("Time Out"), and before the patient leaves the operating room ("Sign Out"). The manual provides suggestions for implementation considering each local environment.[21]

The broader concepts of a learning organization,[22] learning collaboratives,[23,24] and the Framework for Spread[25] have been used effectively to create behavioral changes in health care teams. For example, the Institute for Healthcare Improvement Breakthrough Series Collaboratives have shown improvements in the quality of care for end-of-life and chronic care patients. The collaborative method brings together multiple sites that are similar in a common aim to adapt and spread existing knowledge into practice.[23]

There are also many nationally recognized resources that can be used to prepare health professionals and staff to work in teams and improve quality and safety. See Appendix F for a list of programs and resources for use by frontline staff as well as those that can be useful for staff and faculty development. All the programs and materials are free of charge. The programs range from TeamSTEPPS, a standardized, evidence-based curriculum developed by the US Department of Defense and the Agency for Healthcare Research and Quality to the Veterans Affairs National Quality Scholars Fellowship Program, a two-year interprofessional fellowship program.

Also *see* Appendix F for a list of tools that can be used before and after practice-based interventions to assess the impact of the training on teamwork and collaboration. The first two instruments measure attitudes and perceptions as a result of the TeamSTEPPS training. Although the other tools may require additional validation before being used in research studies, they can be useful for baseline data and pilot studies comparing different tools. Methods available to measure teamwork include self-assessment, peer assessment, 360° evaluations, direct observation, survey of climate and culture, and measurement of outcomes.

Concluding Remarks

In this chapter, we support the implementation of teamwork and collaboration in health care. However, empirical evidence regarding the effectiveness of teamwork and collaboration is not conclusive. A national panel has identified the need to develop metrics to examine the effectiveness of teamwork and interprofessional education in changing behavior in practice and the effects in clinical care. The most effective approach to educate both new and experienced health professionals is yet to be defined.

Ineffective collaboration between physicians, nurses, and other health care practitioners has been associated with poor clinical outcomes and more clinical errors. Assessing and measuring teamwork and collaboration is a matter of continued study.

References

1. Interprofessional Education Collaborative. Team-Based Competencies: Building a Shared Foundation for Education and Clinical Practice. Conference proceedings, Washington, DC, Feb 16–17, 2011. Accessed Oct 18, 2012. https://www.aamc.org/download/186752/data/team-based_competencies.pdf.

2. Estrada CA, et al. Mastering improvement science skills in the new era of quality and safety: The Veterans Affairs National Quality Scholars Program. *J Eval Clin Pract.* 2012 Apr;18(2):508–514.

3. Centers for Medicare & Medicaid Services. Medicaid program; payment adjustment for provider-preventable conditions including health care-acquired conditions. Final rule. *Fed Regist.* 2011 Jun 6;76(108):32816–32838.

4. O'Leary KJ, et al.; for the High Performance Teams and the Hospital of the Future Project Team. Interdisciplinary teamwork in hospitals: A review and practical recommendations for improvement. *J Hosp Med.* 2012 Jan;7(1):48–54.

5. Reeves S, et al. Interprofessional education: Effects on professional practice and health care outcomes. *Cochrane Database Syst Rev.* 2008 Jan 23;(1):CD002213.

6. Reeves S, et al. The effectiveness of interprofessional education: Key findings from a new systematic review. *J Interprof Care.* 2010 May;24(3):230–241.

7. Baker DP, et al. The role of teamwork in the professional education of physicians: Current status and assessment recommendations. *Jt Comm J Qual Patient Saf.* 2005 Apr;31(4):185–202.

8. McPherson K, Headrick L, Moss F. Working and learning together: Good quality care depends on it, but how can we achieve it? *Qual Health Care.* 2001 Dec;10 Suppl 2:i46–i53.

9. Greiner AC, Knebel E; Committee on the Health Professions Education Summit, Institute of Medicine. *Health Professions Education: A Bridge to Quality.* Washington, DC: National Academies Press, 2003.

10. Ladden MD, et al. Educating interprofessional learners for quality, safety and systems improvement. *J Interprof Care.* 2006 Oct;20(5):497–505.

11. Hammick M, et al. A best evidence systematic review of interprofessional education: BEME Guide no. 9. *Med Teach.* 2007 Oct;29(8):735–751.

12. Zwarenstein M, Goldman J, Reeves S. Interprofessional collaboration: Effects of practice-based interventions on professional practice and healthcare outcomes. *Cochrane Database Syst Rev.* 2009 Jul 8;(3):CD000072.

13. Salas E, Gregory ME, King HB. Team training can enhance patient safety—The data, the challenge ahead. *Jt Comm J Qual Patient Saf.* 2011 Aug;37(8):339–340.

14. Weaver SJ, et al. Does teamwork improve performance in the operating room? A multilevel evaluation. *Jt Comm J Qual Patient Saf.* 2010 Mar;36(3):133–142.

15. Weaver SJ, Salas E, King HB. Twelve best practices for team training evaluation in health care. *Jt Comm J Qual Patient Saf.* 2011 Aug;37(8):341–349.

16. Spector JM, et al. Improving quality of care for maternal and newborn health: Prospective pilot study of the WHO safe childbirth checklist program. *PLoS One.* Epub 2012 May 16.

17. Koll BS, et al. The CLABs collaborative: A regionwide effort to improve the quality of care in hospitals. *Jt Comm J Qual Patient Saf.* 2008 Dec;34(12):713–723.

18. Kim JS, Holtom P, Vigen C. Reduction of catheter-related bloodstream infections through the use of a central venous line bundle: Epidemiologic and economic consequences. *Am J Infect Control.* 2011 Oct;39(8):640–646.

19. Haynes AB, et al.; Safe Surgery Saves Lives Study Group. A surgical safety checklist to reduce morbidity and mortality in a global population. *N Engl J Med.* 2009 Jan 29;360(5):491–499.

20. Pronovost P, et al. An intervention to decrease catheter-related bloodstream infections in the ICU. *N Engl J Med.* 2006 Dec 28;355(26):2725–2732. Erratum in: *N Engl J Med.* 2007 Jun 21;356(25):2660.

21. World Health Organization. Implementation Manual: WHO Surgical Safety Checklist. World Alliance for Patient Safety. 2008. Accessed Oct 18, 2012. http://www.who.int/patientsafety/safesurgery/tools_resources/SSSL_Manual_finalJun08.pdf.

22. Senge PM. *The Fifth Discipline: The Art and Practice of the Learning Organization,* rev. ed. New York: Currency Doubleday, 2006.

23. Kilo CM. A framework for collaborative improvement: Lessons from the Institute for Healthcare Improvement's Breakthrough Series. *Qual Manag Health Care.* 1998 Sep;6(4):1–13.

24. Wilson T, Berwick DM, Cleary PD. What do collaborative improvement projects do? Experience from seven countries. *Jt Comm J Qual Saf.* 2003 Feb;29(2):85–93.

25. Massoud MR, et al. *A Framework for Spread: From Local Improvements to System-Wide Change.* IHI Innovation Series white paper. Cambridge, MA: Institute for Healthcare Improvement, 2006.

Chapter 9

APPLYING PRACTICE-BASED LEARNING AND IMPROVEMENT

Mary A. Dolansky, Mamta K. Singh, Brook Watts, Renée H. Lawrence, Eugene C. Nelson, Paul B. Batalden, William H. Edwards, Carlos A. Estrada, Mark E. Splaine

The first steps toward clinical improvement might indeed feel like small ones, as the task is large. In a system as vast and complex as modern health care, we might struggle to imagine how small tests of local change can meaningfully alter outcomes beyond the front door of one's organization. But larger changes are indeed built up from mutually supportive smaller ones, and improvement methods appropriate to microsystem levels of care can be effectively applied at the mesosystem and macrosystem levels as well.

This chapter presents advanced applications of improvement as developed in increasingly complex and inclusive systems of care. We review two case studies that illustrate the forms of knowledge and action we have previously explored, in contexts that extend local implementation to regional and national domains. In the first case, we describe the framework known as the patient-centered medical home or primary care medical home (*see* Sidebar 9-1, page 110) and a specific effort to implement this framework in the US Department of Veterans Affairs (VA)—specifically, in its Veterans Health Administration (VHA) health care facilities—that is illustrative of interprofessional efforts to accomplish practice-based learning and improvement. The case highlights key moments in the history of the patient-centered medical home, the opportunities to include practice-based learning and improvement into patient-centered medical home goals, and the integration of patient-centered medical home and practice-based learning and improvement into resident and nurse practitioner learner training.

The second case draws on a national inpatient care collaborative of neonatal intensive care units (NICUs)—the Vermont Oxford Network (VON). Since 1988 this network of NICUs has been improving care in local settings and across the network using the principles of practice-based learning and improvement. This case highlights the use of an international registry that includes more than 900 NICUs from 28 countries. The registry data are based on the four quadrants of the Clinical Value Compass—clinical, functional, satisfaction, and costs. The VON sites share evidence-based practice, systems thinking, collaborative learning, and interventions for improvement. Throughout the chapter, we recognize the hands-on learning that proceeds in parallel with health care improvement—the learning that directs and refines improvement work.

Case 1: VHA Practice-Based Learning and Improvement to Facilitate Team-Based Care

Background: The Need for Transformation

Addressing the challenges and opportunities created by chronic disease management for both primary and specialty care services necessitated and continues to necessitate visions, frameworks, strategies, and tools that enable practice transformation. When viewed this way, the patient-centered medical home and practice-based learning and improvement (or quality improvement in general) are natural partners. Indeed, many of the driving forces that culminated in the patient-centered medical home

Sidebar 9-1. Patient-Centered Medical Home: Why Now?

The reemergence of the model known as the patient-centered medical home or primary care medical home, a 40-year-old concept that is gaining both medical and political traction, is not entirely coincidental. With the growing number of patients who are older than 65 years of age, there has been an increase in chronic diseases in the patient population, which has led to an increase in health care costs, with up to 17% of the gross domestic product of the United States spent on health care. Coupling these challenges with the lack of access to primary care and the decreasing number of clinicians going into primary care, the US health care delivery system is in need of a transformative culture change. The patient-centered medical home model is being reintroduced today because it provides an opportunity to realign priorities and redeploy resources to ensure that patients have access to high-quality primary care.

In addition, The Joint Commission primary care medical home model is based on the Agency for Healthcare Research and Quality's definition of a medical home, which describes a medical home as a model of primary care that includes patient-centered care, comprehensive care, coordinated care, access to care, and a systems-based approach to quality and safety. The Joint Commission was scheduled to start certification of primary care medical homes in 2013. More information and resources can be found at http://www.jointcommission.org/assets/1/18/Joint_Commission_PCMH_model.pdf and http://www.jointcommission.org/assets/1/18/PCMH.pdf.

models can be summarized under practice-based learning and improvement change concepts such as those addressed in Chapter 6 (*see* Figures 6-2 and 6-4 on pages 77 and 80). Specific examples are improvement of work flow, optimization of staff, enhancement of the customer relationship, management of variation, and design of systems to avoid mistakes and focus on the service.

In the Safety Net Medical Home Initiative put forth in 2009 by Qualis Health and the MacColl Institute for Healthcare Innovation (*see* Sidebar 9-2 below), it was clearly outlined that for patient-centered medical home practices to be successful, they need to "choose and use a formal model for quality improvement."[1] Aligning both

practice-based learning and improvement and the patient-centered medical home would create an interface that furthers the goals of both frameworks. Planning a baseline and then an outcomes-based Clinical Value Compass will crystallize opportunities and ways to align forces to navigate quality outcomes, use panel management to enhance access and care coordination, and recognize the importance of engaging all stakeholders within the context of continuous and team-based healing relationships. This case study provides a better sense of the impact of these change concepts and the general common trends for the emergence and momentum of the patient-centered medical home.

Our four main objectives for this case are to do the following:

1. Highlight key moments in the history of the patient-centered medical home and the VHA Patient Aligned Care Team (PACT) that enabled (or, rather, reenabled) its momentum.
2. Discuss the clinical setting and the location of the work.
3. Suggest major opportunities for how practice-based learning and improvement can further patient-centered medical home goals and vision (and vice versa).
4. Provide suggestions to maximize creating and sustaining patient-centered medical home / VHA PACT as a learning environment.

Sidebar 9-2. About Qualis and MacColl

Qualis Health is a nonprofit health care quality improvement organization dedicated to improving the quality of health care delivery and health outcomes for individuals and populations across the United States. Further information about Qualis Health is available online at http://www.qualishealth.org.

The MacColl Institute for Healthcare Innovation serves as the national program office for the Robert Wood Johnson Foundation's program for improving chronic illness care. The goal is to develop, evaluate, and disseminate innovations in health care delivery by bridging the worlds of research and clinical care. For further information, visit the MacColl Institute website at http://www.improvingchroniccare.org.

History of the VHA Patient-Centered Medical Home

The patient-centered medical home is a model of care that applies a comprehensive team approach to patient care on the basis of a fundamental relationship between a patient and his or her main health care provider. The primary provider guides relevant team members necessary to provide the full range of care for the patient. The patient-centered medical home in many ways revisits the "tradition" of relationship-based care between providers and their patient with the promise of "tomorrow" in the form of information technology (electronic medical records, registries, and various modes of virtual health care).

The American Academy of Pediatrics introduced the term *medical home* in 1967 in an effort to improve care of children with special needs. Initially it was used to describe a single source of medical information about a patient, but its meaning gradually grew to include a partnership approach with families to provide primary health care that is accessible, family-centered, coordinated, comprehensive, continuous, compassionate, and culturally effective.[1]

The World Health Organization (WHO) convened an international conference on primary health care in 1978 at Alma-Ata in the Soviet Union and defined some basic tenets of the medical home and the important role of primary care.[2] Specifically, the Alma-Ata conference report states that "primary health care is the key"[2(p. 3)] to obtaining adequate "health, which is a state of complete physical, mental and social wellbeing, and not merely the absence of disease or infirmity."[2(p. 2)]

These WHO concepts were later included in a report issued in the 1990s by the Institute of Medicine, which mentioned the "medical home."[3] This report influenced many disciplines, and in particular, the medical home concept began to appear in the family medicine literature. In 2002 family medicine physicians looked at how to develop a strategy to transform and renew the discipline of family medicine to meet the needs of patients in a changing health care environment. This examination resulted in the Future of Family Medicine Project, which states that every American should have a "Personal Medical Home" through which all individuals—regardless of age, sex, race, or socioeconomic status—receive their acute, chronic, and preventive medical services.[4]

Another important initiative in further defining the core principles of the patient-centered medical home was the Chronic Care Model developed by Edward Wagner. Studies using the Chronic Care Model have demonstrated improvement in the quality of care and reduction in cost for patients with chronic diseases.[5] These studies led to the 2007 publication of the "Joint Principles of the Patient-Centered Medical Home," which defined the seven core principles of a medical home and was endorsed by the American Academy of Family Physicians, American Academy of Pediatrics, American College of Physicians, and American Osteopathic Association.[6] The coming together of these organizations was as inspirational as the seven core features they proposed.

The original seven core principles of the patient-centered medical home are as follows.[6] Note that the original language in the document included the term "personal physician." In contemporary medical home models, the "personal physician" role is expanded to include nurse practitioners, physician assistants, and advanced practice nurses.

1. **Personal Physician:** Each patient has an ongoing relationship with a personal provider trained to provide first contact and continuous, comprehensive care.

2. **Physician-Directed Medical Practice:** The personal physician leads a team of individuals at the practice level who collectively take responsibility for the ongoing care of patients.

3. **Whole Person Orientation:** The personal physician is responsible for providing all the patient's health care needs or taking responsibility for appropriately arranging care with other qualified professionals.

4. **Coordinated Care:** Care is coordinated and/or integrated across all elements of the complex health care system (for example, subspecialty care, hospitals, home health agencies, nursing homes) and the patient's community (for example, family, public and private community-based services). Care is facilitated

by registries, information technology, health information exchange, and other means to ensure that patients get the indicated care when and where they need and want it in a culturally and linguistically appropriate manner.

5. **Quality and Safety:** Quality and safety are hallmarks of the medical home, as demonstrated in the following ways:

— Providers advocate for their patients to support the attainment of optimal, patient-centered outcomes that are defined by a care planning process driven by a compassionate, robust partnership among physicians, patients, and patients' families.

— Evidence-based medicine and clinical decision-support tools guide decision making.

— Physicians in the practice accept accountability for continuous quality improvement through voluntary engagement in performance measurement and improvement.

— Information technology is used appropriately to support optimal patient care, performance measurement, patient education, and enhanced communication.

— Patients and families participate in quality improvement activities at the practice level.

6. **Greater Access to Care:** Enhanced access is available through systems such as open scheduling, expanded hours, and new options for communication between patients and their physician and practice staff.

7. **Payment Reform:** The payment system is changed in a way that recognizes the added value provided to patients who have a patient-centered medical home. For example, it should reflect the value of physician and nonphysician staff patient-centered care management work that falls outside of the face-to-face visit. It should support adoption of and use of health information technology for quality improvement. It should allow for additional payments for achieving measurable and continuous quality improvements.

These core principles have served as the foundation for many institutions, including the VHA, as they redesign their primary delivery systems (*see* Sidebar 9-3, below).

Other patient-centered medical home resources include the American College of Physicians (https://www.medicalhomebuilder.org/home), the National Committee for Quality Assurance (http://www.ncqa.org/tabid/631/Default.aspx), The Joint Commission (http://www.jointcommission.org/accreditation/pchi.aspx), the Agency for Healthcare Research and Quality (http://pcmh.ahrq.gov/portal/server.pt/community/pcmh__home), the Patient-Centered Primary Care Collaborative (http://www.pcpcc.net/), and the VHA (http://www.va.gov/primarycare/pcmh/).

Clinical Setting: The Location of the Work

The PACT engages patients in a more active role to manage their health care rather than being advised what to do through a provider-centered system. The VHA PACT integrates the patient-centered medical home core principles but also includes other core principles as its foundation: patient-driven, team-based, efficient, comprehensive, coordinated, communication-oriented, and continuous. It is expected that the VHA PACT will result in improved quality, greater veteran satisfaction, and cost savings from decreased hospital visits and fewer readmissions through patient-focused care. This model is meant to focus on all patients receiving

---

Sidebar 9-3. Making a PACT

The Veterans Health Administration (VHA) implemented the patient-centered medical home model in 2010. The patient-centered medical home is known in the VHA system as PACT (Patient Aligned Care Team). The goals of the PACT are to provide access to primary care, seamless coordination of care between VHA providers and non-VHA providers, and patient-centered coordinated care using interdisciplinary teams. The PACT care team considers all aspects of patient health, with an emphasis on prevention and health promotion. At the center of the care team is the patient (and the patient's family members). Health care professionals include a primary care provider, nurse care manager, clinical associate, and administrative clerk.

VHA primary care, which is known to be 80% to 90% of the enrolled veteran patient population.

The Practice Environment: Integration of Practice-Based Learning and Improvement into the Patient-Centered Medical Home

Successful and sustainable applications of quality improvement to clinical care benefit from team-based approaches. Thus, there is the potential for an important synergy among efforts to engage frontline clinical staff in practice-based learning and improvement and the spread of the patient-centered medical home model. In particular, the patient-centered medical home focus on interdisciplinary engagement may be of critical importance to the successful integration of practice-based learning and improvement into team-based models of care. Given that one of the primary potential benefits of the patient-centered medical home is an impact on quality across the spectrum of key quality-of-care components—including safety, effectiveness, efficiency, patient-centeredness, timeliness, and equity—the stakes are high to demonstrate successful improvement efforts in this and other new models of care. However, challenges to the integration of practice-based learning and improvement into the patient-centered medical home exist, including the potential lack of tools to facilitate interdisciplinary team-based efforts to improve care and the potential lack of quality metrics to measure team-based care. Efforts to address these challenges will be critical to ensure that the improvement potential of the patient-centered medical home and integration of practice-based learning and improvement is realized.

Challenge 1: Tools to Support Integration of the Patient-Centered Medical Home and Practice-Based Learning and Improvement

Clinical improvement efforts often focus on improving care for a group of patients through application of a national guideline as a surrogate measurement for evidence-based care. With this approach, the improvement work tends to shift from a one-on-one relationship between a patient and a provider to a broader team-based approach to enhance care for a group (or "panel")

of patients. The emphasis on panel management approaches is most evident for chronic diseases, such as diabetes, heart failure, and hepatitis C. As interdisciplinary teams have developed new approaches to chronic disease management, it is increasingly apparent that efficient and effective management of chronic diseases necessitates tools that meet a particular set of needs for the patient-centered medical home team. Specifically, management of chronic diseases is an empiric, iterative process, which requires multiple clinical evaluations as well as frequent adjustments of pharmacologic therapies, repetitive laboratory testing, and innovative behavior change strategies. These repetitive clinical processes pose a significant challenge for the patient and the patient-centered medical home team. To increase usefulness of face-to-face visits and maximize effectiveness of between-visit care, teams need tools that provide accurate, timely, flexible, and accessible information about the health status of a patient or a group of patients. In addition, tools to facilitate panel management approaches may be particularly relevant, given the new emphasis on non-face-to-face services, including telehealth programs and online interactions between patients and care teams via e-mail or websites. Interprofessional tools include measurement of and training for advanced teamwork and communication skills and systems thinking that many health care practitioners did not receive in their professional education.

The increasing shift toward use of electronic health records (EHRs) has made it far easier to extract data on a large number of patients, thus creating the opportunity to easily construct tools to facilitate improvement approaches for panel management. Specifically, as the EHR has continued to evolve, frontline clinicians and quality management staff have become increasingly engaged by the potential of fostering local registry approaches for data obtained within the context of routine clinical management. Logically, this shift may be a result of the propagation of performance measurement and other benchmarking approaches, such as those of The Joint Commission and Medicare, which require clinicians, hospitals, or health care systems to be able to produce information on groups of patients in a low-cost and timely fashion (for example, the percentage of diabetic patients who have achieved target blood pressure). In the context of the patient-centered medical home, the successful application of practice-based learning and improvement using approaches to manage panels of patients requires addressing the following key questions:

1. Do the appropriate tools exist to summarize information on panels of patients for members of the patient-centered medical home team?

2. Who is charged with ensuring that the panel management data meet the needs of the team for ongoing quality improvement activities? For example, if a patient-centered medical home team initiates an effort to improve influenza vaccination in its patient population, who ensures that the appropriate data are available for the team?

3. Who ensures that team-based improvement activities align with the goals of the local care environment and health care system and vice versa?

Health care systems and care environments that successfully address these questions may be optimally positioned to ensure that integration of the patient-centered medical home and practice-based learning and improvement leads to enhanced clinical care and improved outcomes for patients. However, the success of these new tools requires information technology development processes that embrace the roles of interdisciplinary team members and recognize that clinical processes of care are exceedingly local. The importance of flexibility at all levels, including measurement, display, and applications of electronic tools to support patient-centered medical home improvement efforts, cannot be overstated. "One-size-fits-all" solutions will not effectively meet the needs of interdisciplinary teams in successful and sustainable integration of practice-based learning and improvement into the care environment. Information technology development teams that embrace all frontline clinical stakeholders, not just physicians, will be critical to the success of these endeavors.

Challenge 2: Development of Team-Based Improvement Outcomes

After tools are in place to support the integration of practice-based learning and improvement and the patient-centered medical home, a second challenge to successful integration is the development of measurements that support team-based improvement efforts. The Clinical Value Compass can be used to guide the choice of outcomes that include clinical indicators, functional status, satisfaction, and cost (*see* Chapter 4 and Appendix A). The continuity and teamwork provided by the patient-centered medical home has an advantage over traditional ambulatory care in that the team can monitor and support minor improvements in patients' outcomes. The following is an example of how traditional ways of measuring outcomes may not adequately capture key components of patient care that reflect the work of interdisciplinary team members:

A particular patient has poorly controlled hypertension. His primary care provider has seen him regularly over several years and made recommendations for dietary changes and medication adherence; however, the patient has not shown clinical improvement between the three-month appointments. A patient-centered medical home model is implemented, and this patient is identified in a panel of high-risk hypertensive patients to be targeted for intervention by the patient-centered medical home nurse case manager. She calls the patient daily to check his home blood pressure reading and repeatedly emphasizes dietary changes. Over many weeks, the nurse case manager cultivates a strong rapport with the patient. The patient makes small improvements over time in his diet and is more adherent to his medical regimen, although at his next primary care visit, he still has not achieved target blood pressure control.

Did this patient receive quality care? Intuitively, the answer is yes. Yet within the context of many existing models of care and the current way we measure outcomes, the answer is obviously no. Most traditional models still focus on capturing a key component of evidence-based care, such as a specific blood pressure target or a cholesterol or hemoglobin A1c result. In the case example, it seems clear that team-based care has improved the overall quality of the patient's care and likely his long-term outcomes. However, the usual outcome (achieving a target blood pressure) has not been met. In particular, this type of traditional outcome does not appear to reflect the contributions of the nonphysician team members to the care of the patient.

What is the alternative to the traditional disease-based process and outcome measures? In the context of patient-centered medical home and practice-based learning and improvement integration, it may be uniquely important to designate individual team members as responsible for documentation of respective components of additional outcome measures such as those in the Clinical Value Compass. In the example, rather than solely measuring the short-term outcome of blood pressure target in a patient with a long history of uncontrolled hypertension (clinical indicators), other measurement possibilities under the functional status and satisfaction categories of the Clinical Value Compass can include the following:

- Number of non-face-to-face contacts between patient and care team and satisfaction with these encounters
- Documentation of patient understanding of dietary information delivered by nonphysician team member
- Documentation of objective assessment of self-management skills, taking into consideration patient preferences, health literacy, depression, and cognitive function

Discussion of how the work of the patient-centered medical home nurse and other team members contributes to the work of the primary care provider and reduces costs (and value) is particularly relevant, given the popularity and expansion of Medicare and other pay-for-performance programs. Financial incentives from Medicare and other programs for provision of "quality care" may benefit the primary care provider directly, despite the contributions of other team members, unless other strategies are specifically made. Specific efforts to align pay-for-performance metrics with the goals of the patient-centered medical home will be critical to the sustainability of these efforts.

The Learning Environment: Integrating Practice-Based Learning and Improvement into the Patient-Centered Medical Home

This evolution to the patient-centered medical home provides a unique opportunity for interdisciplinary student learning, particularly for resident and nurse practitioner education. The Veterans Health Administration and its partnerships with affiliated academic institutions provide the largest education and training effort for health professionals in the United States. In 2010 more than 115,000 trainees received some or all of their clinical training in the VHA. Almost all Veterans Affairs medical centers have affiliation agreements with most accredited medical schools (including osteopathic medicine); in addition, 40 other health professions have affiliation agreements with more than 1,200 colleges and universities. Thus, the VHA supports five Centers of Excellence in Primary Care. These centers are charged with the development, implementation, and evaluation of an interprofessional curriculum to train nurse practitioners and residents in the PACT model.[7]

The organizing framework for the curriculum includes the following four elements:

1. Shared decision making (to support patient-centered approaches)
2. Sustained relationships (to promote longitudinal patient care relationships)
3. Interprofessional collaboration (to support teamwork)
4. Performance improvement (to promote continual quality improvement)

Specific to practice-based learning and improvement, trainees attend sessions on the foundations of quality improvement, quality improvement methodology, tools, and systems thinking. At the Louis Stokes Cleveland VA Medical Center, trainees (along with patient-centered medical home staff) receive Six Sigma yellow belt certification, use registries to assess panel data, and integrate teamwork and collaboration. Teams of residents and nurse practitioner students meet twice a week to review their panel of patients and identify areas for improvement. The trainees are mentored by the PACT teams and the clinic nurses who have expertise in panel management.

The trainees examine key clinical indicators and extract panels of patients who are not meeting their expectations. Trainees learn to move from individual-centered care to systems thinking to identify a systems improvement. After an area of improvement is identified, the trainees, as a part of an interdisciplinary team, develop and implement a quality improvement project, such as the example shown in Sidebar 9-4, below. The experience ends with a presentation of the project and a manuscript using the Standards for Quality Improvement Reporting Excellence (SQUIRE) guidelines (see Appendix H for further information about the SQUIRE guidelines).

This unique blending of practice-based learning and improvement into daily care helps learners integrate continual improvement into their routine clinical decision making. Using the PACT as a learning environment, learners not only do their work but also improve their work. An appreciation builds that practice-based learning and improvement is a part of the process and not a separate step.

Conclusion

If skills and tools are truly learned, they become a natural extension of the provider's and learner's approach. An environment that provides the resources for practice-based learning and improvement is needed to ensure that practice-based learning and improvement is integrated into health care providers' work—rather than stopping actual health care to look for ways to practice or apply practice-based learning and improvement

competencies—and the patient-centered medical home has created an opportunity to do just that.

Case 2: The Vermont Oxford Network's Use of Clinical Value Compass Thinking for Learning and Benchmarking for Improvement
Background: The Need for Innovation
In the 1980s, when physician and author William H. Edwards was medical director of Dartmouth-Hitchcock Medical Center's intensive care nursery (ICN), he had a dream "to achieve the best outcomes in the world." The means to such a vision, however, were not immediately apparent. Certainly, members of the ICN staff were talented, hardworking individuals and were committed to clinical excellence. But how could these professionals be effectively directed to achievement of "best-in-the-world" outcomes, and indeed, how might such outcomes even be identified? Two strategic interventions have proven particularly valuable to actualize this vision: the creation of a registry of ICN outcomes known as the Vermont Oxford Network (VON) and implementation (both locally and internationally, in the context of this larger network) of value compass techniques.

Clinical Setting: Location of the Work
Established in 1988, the VON is now an international clinical association of more than 900 neonatal intensive care units (NICUs) in 28 countries.[8] The network brings together diverse practice sites in terms of size, patient sociodemographic composition, geographic

---

Sidebar 9-4. Quality Improvement Project Example

An example of a quality improvement project developed by a practice-based learning and improvement team is a facility priority project of improving diabetes care for women. Although the project aim is to identify 95% of the team's female patients with HbA1c < 9, and the intervention is the implementation of motivational interviewing, students are encouraged to tailor a new topic to meet their needs. After the team has conducted a microsystem assessment, a student on the team could choose, for example, to implement insulin titration or add mental health services. Challenges of integrating transient members in existing practice-based learning and improvement teams are overcome by ensuring that the project is not dependent on any one trainee, non-face-to-face means of communication are used, trainees are educated and skilled at data acquisition from panel registries, and team training is provided to leverage interdisciplinary team members to facilitate the success of the team.

location, academic affiliation, and urban/ community settings. VON members share core values concerning the delivery of high-quality care, participate in educational and research activities, and collect standardized data on infants of very low birth weight (VLBW)—that is, infants weighing less than 1,500 grams at birth. Sites foster shared habits of evidence-based practice, systems thinking, collaborative learning, and changing for improvement.

Participants collaborate in original research and in dissemination of evidence-based best practices.[9] Members can also participate in annual educational events and in multiyear clinical learning collaboratives; since 1995, more than 300 teams have participated in collaboratives. A major VON process is the collection of data (benchmarking, as described in detail in Chapter 5) on clinical processes and outcomes in all member NICUs. To realize the dream of optimized clinical care, VON practitioners can use real-time data to answer central questions such as "Which NICUs have the best outcomes in the world, and what are they doing to achieve these superior results?"

Outcomes measurement is thus central to the VON's research and improvement mission. From the outset, the network developed standard metrics to define vital clinical outcomes— mortality and morbidity associated with premature birth. To expand the scope of this outcomes database and to generate balanced measures that are relevant to families, clinical teams, institutions, and society, the VON has embraced the methods and modeling of the Clinical Value Compass.

Application of Clinical Value Compass Concepts

The Clinical Value Compass (described in detail in Chapter 4) has been used in the ICN at the Dartmouth-Hitchcock Medical Center since 1992 for infants and has facilitated clarification, monitoring, and achievement of specific outcomes that matter most to premature infants and their families (*see* Figure 9-1, page 118). In 2004 the VON launched the "Your Ideal NICU" program, which was designed to dramatically improve care

in NICUs at 12 health care organizations. An interdisciplinary task force designed, tested, and implemented a Clinical Value Compass approach for VLBW infants. The intention was to pilot test the value compass with a subset of participating sites and then refine it for future use by all VON members. The Joint Commission has expanded the VON model of sharing outcomes by sharing a Web-based performance improvement template for institutions to use to accelerate change. The Joint Commission Center for Transforming Healthcare provides a Targeted Solutions Tool™ that guides staff through three performance improvement projects: hand hygiene, handoff communication, and wrong site surgery (for details, *see* http:// www.centerfortransforminghealthcare.org/about/ default.aspx). The VON and Joint Commission models provide valuable resources that will have an impact on accelerating improvement.

Methods: How It Works

The VON VLBW Clinical Value Compass (for infants 500–1,500 grams) includes the four conventional quadrants (clinical, functional, satisfaction, and costs). Each participating NICU collects and submits data on the basis of written protocols. Data sets are sent to a central VON location for analysis and distribution. Sites receive an annual feedback report that describes local performance in absolute and relative terms—that is, in comparison to other participating NICUs—as follows:

- Clinical outcomes data for VLBW infants reflect mortality, morbidity, and treatment complications experienced during the NICU stay. Standard operational definitions are used to determine the presence or absence of clinical conditions and the values of clinical measures.

- Functional outcomes for premature infants are assessed using a special "transitions" survey completed by parents a few weeks after discharge. The survey queries basic activities of both baby and family in the context of the potentially challenging transition to home. The short-term functional assessment will be supplemented by intermediate (age 6 months

Figure 9-1. Original Very Low Birth Weight Infant Clinical Value Compass Developed by Dartmouth-Hitchcock Medical Center Intensive Care Nursery

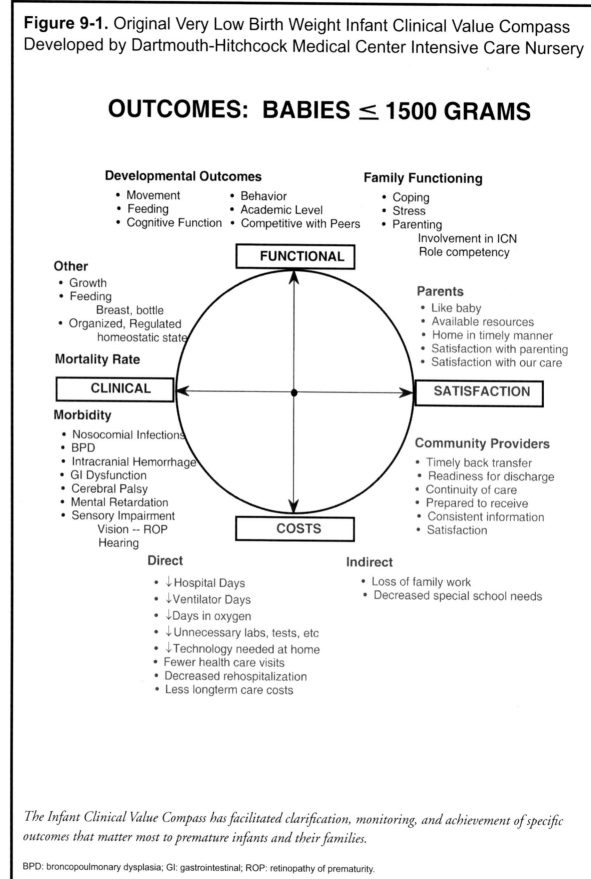

OUTCOMES: BABIES ≤ 1500 GRAMS

Developmental Outcomes
- Movement
- Behavior
- Feeding
- Academic Level
- Cognitive Function
- Competitive with Peers

Family Functioning
- Coping
- Stress
- Parenting
  Involvement in ICN
  Role competency

Other
- Growth
- Feeding
  Breast, bottle
- Organized, Regulated
  homeostatic state

Mortality Rate

Parents
- Like baby
- Available resources
- Home in timely manner
- Satisfaction with parenting
- Satisfaction with our care

FUNCTIONAL

CLINICAL

SATISFACTION

COSTS

Morbidity
- Nosocomial Infections
- BPD
- Intracranial Hemorrhage
- GI Dysfunction
- Cerebral Palsy
- Mental Retardation
- Sensory Impairment
  Vision -- ROP
  Hearing

Community Providers
- Timely back transfer
- Readiness for discharge
- Continuity of care
- Prepared to receive
- Consistent information
- Satisfaction

Direct
- ↓Hospital Days
- ↓Ventilator Days
- ↓Days in oxygen
- ↓Unnecessary labs, tests, etc
- ↓Technology needed at home
- Fewer health care visits
- Decreased rehospitalization
- Less longterm care costs

Indirect
- Loss of family work
- Decreased special school needs

The Infant Clinical Value Compass has facilitated clarification, monitoring, and achievement of specific outcomes that matter most to premature infants and their families.

BPD: broncopoulmonary dysplasia; GI: gastrointestinal; ROP: retinopathy of prematurity.

Source: Reproduced with permission from The Dartmouth Institute for Health Policy and Clinical Practice (TDI).

to 2 years postdischarge) and longer-term outcomes.

- Satisfaction assessment focuses on parental perceptions of care by NICU staff and on perceptions of their own participation in this care. Feedback is collected through an Internet-based survey (http://www.howsyourbaby.com, available only at participating institutions) that was specifically designed for parents of preterm infants receiving NICU care.

- The VON Clinical Value Compass defines two cost metrics: Length of NICU stay is used as a proxy for direct medical care costs, whereas parents' evaluation of overall financial burden (including time lost from work and other opportunity costs) serves as a marker for indirect social costs.

Displays and Utility: What It Looks Like and How It Is Used

For more than two decades, clinicians and staff at ICNs have used the Clinical Value Compass shown in Figure 9-1 to do the following:

- Clarify general goals and specify important outcomes
- Set priorities for improving results
- Communicate with patients, colleagues, and other stakeholders about achievements in high-quality, safe, cost-effective care

Use of value compass thinking has enabled ICN caregivers to develop specific improvement projects in all four quadrants:

- **Clinical:** minimizing infants' exposures to loud noises, decreasing the rate of nosocomial infections, and lowering the incidence of chronic lung disease
- **Functional:** improving families' feelings of security and competency in postdischarge baby care
- **Satisfaction:** promoting parents' self-perception as "caregiving partners" with NICU staff and improving parent evaluations of care provided by NICU staff
- **Costs:** decreasing lengths of stay, reducing unnecessary diagnostic tests, and facilitating early discharge to infants' homes or community hospitals

The Clinical Value Compass permits expansion of outcome measures available for comparative benchmarking and improvement. "Your Ideal NICU" program activities that are based in part on value compass thinking yielded dramatic results at a number of sites. Improvements have been documented in such domains as parent–infant bonding, effective use of evidence-based protocols, coordinated handoffs for incoming and outgoing infants, and decreased nosocomial infections.

To introduce participating centers to value compass methods, the VON has sponsored a six-session distance learning program facilitated by a Web communication company. The first session introduces the Clinical Value Compass, and the next four sessions "circle" its four points. Between sessions, participants engage in "translational homework," adapting general ideas and methods to their own clinical settings, constructing local value compasses, and selecting key outcomes in each quadrant for analysis and intervention. In the final collective session, individual sites present their progress reports and discuss specific follow-up projects to sustain and extend initial improvements.

Further Applications and Implementation

The larger network of VON practices continues to document its successes. Some of these initiatives have led to substantial and measurable improvements in outcomes related to nosocomial infections, noise exposure, and length of stay.[9] Participating institutions may have different priority improvement projects ongoing to maintain the "best in the world" vision, or participating institutions can be part of a clinical learning collaborative.[10]

The National Quality Forum (NQF), a not-for-profit organization that sets national priorities for performance improvement, has endorsed several of the VON measures.[11] Examples of VON measures that are now NQF priorities include the following:

- *NQF # 0303. Late sepsis or meningitis in neonates (risk-adjusted).* Percentage of infants born at the hospital, whose birth weight is between 401 and 1,500 grams *or* whose gestational age is between 22 weeks 0 days and 29 weeks 6 days with late sepsis or meningitis with one or more of the following criteria: bacterial pathogen, coagulase negative *Staphylococcus*, or fungal infection.

- *NQF # 0304. Late sepsis or meningitis in Very Low Birth Weight (VLBW) neonates (risk-adjusted).* Standardized rate and standardized morbidity ratio for nosocomial bacterial infection after day 3 of life for very low birth weight infants, including infants with birth weights between 401 and 1,500 grams and infants whose gestational age is between 22 and 29 weeks.

- *NQF # 0481. First temperature measured within one hour of admission to the NICU.* Percentage of NICU admissions with a birth weight of 501 to 1,500 grams with a first temperature taken within one hour of NICU admission.

- *NQF # 0482. First NICU Temperature < 36° Centigrade.* Percentage of all NICU admissions with a birth weight of 501 to 1,500 grams whose first temperature was measured within one hour of admission to the NICU and was below 36° Celsius.

- *NQF # 0483. Proportion of infants 22 to 29 weeks gestation screened for retinopathy of prematurity.* Proportion of infants at 22 to 29 weeks gestation who were in the reporting hospital at the postnatal age recommended for retinopathy of prematurity (ROP) screening by

the American Academy of Pediatrics and who received a retinal examination for ROP prior to discharge.

- *NQF # 0484. Proportion of infants 22 to 29 weeks gestation treated with surfactant who are treated within 2 hours of birth.* Number of infants at 22 to 29 weeks gestation who were treated with surfactant within two hours of birth.

Collaboratives have shown that using the VON data set and a structured approach for quality improvement decreased NICUs' nosocomial infection rates, improved respiratory practices, and increased survival.[12–14]

Challenges and Solutions

In 2011, at a VON national meeting on Collaborative Improvement Networks, the challenges to maintain the network were summarized.[15] Table 9-1 (below) also provides successful strategies that other micro- or macrosystems could apply.

Reflections on Advanced Applications of Practice-Based Learning and Improvement

What can we learn from these two case studies? What common themes are relevant to clinicians

Table 9-1. Challenges and Strategies for Collaborative Improvement Networks

Challenges	Successful Strategies
How to organize and support the vision of a worldwide community of practice	• Support regional, organizational, state, and national collaboratives. • Develop and freely share resources and access to data. • Sponsor improvement venues that can be accessed worldwide.
How to provide value and support to both individual centers and regional, organizational, state, and national collaboratives	• Provide special reports for established groups for comparative outcome data. • Demonstrate value of comparative data from a larger "universe" of neonatal providers. • Invite leaders of collaboratives to participate (without charge) and freely use learning developed in neonatal intensive care unit quality improvement collaboratives.
How to maintain resources sufficient to meet vision (financial, organization structure, personnel, technical, intellectual, leadership, expert faculty)	• Provide value to participants. • Keep basic membership affordable (database, annual meeting, quality congress). • Offer options for participation at various levels (costs). • Take advantage of synergy among initiatives.

in their own daily work of patient care, practice-based learning and improvement, and professional development? Those examples of application of improvement methods and principles depict the same tools and concepts that have been explored throughout the text. Although our examples include a variety of settings, the universal applications of improvement methods and principles are consistent. The following several points warrant specific consideration:

- *Innovative approaches to data collection must be built into daily care processes.* Proper measurement of clinical processes and outcomes requires not only technical expertise but also tireless ingenuity. Successful implementation of both the PACT and VON initiatives required capturing new data streams, in real time, from both patients and clinicians, and this work was facilitated by the Clinical Value Compass outcomes. Novel data collection and user-friendly display strategies had to be designed, tested, and *coordinated with mainstream data-gathering activities,* and health care providers needed to be trained in understanding and using these data sources to facilitate successful improvement.

- *Consideration of outcomes must be balanced and inclusive.* Both the VON and PACT cases remind us that illness and health are not defined simply in terms of the target patient's clinical parameters but that they extend to functional, psychological, and economic experiences of all participants, including parents and community caregivers. Systems thinking and the Clinical Value Compass build such multidimensionality into both daily care and longer-term strategic planning.

- *Increased transparency is a fact of life to be embraced (rather than resisted) in the evolving health care system.* As discussed in Chapter 1, evidence-based metrics are increasingly monitored by employers, regulators, payers, and the public, and this trend will certainly continue in the foreseeable future. Transparency can be turned to collective advantage by individual clinicians and entire health systems in the work of health care

improvement. At the VON, collective data sharing permits comparative benchmarking to achieve better outcomes across participating sites. In the VHA PACT, similar reporting of systemwide outcomes for panels of patients permits dissemination of best strategies for care.

- *Practice-based learning is built into the work itself.* Adult learners in general, and maturing practitioners in particular, learn best (and learn continuously) through an active and iterative process that includes self-generation of ideas, thoughtful implementation of test interventions, careful assessment (including quantitative measurement) of specific consequences, and regular reflection on the process itself. These are indeed the same activities that support clinical improvement work at both microsystem and macrosystem levels. Through processes of increasingly refined trial and error, or trial and success, dedicated practitioners in the VON collaborative and the VHA PACT are learning in the field how to improve primary care, how to raise the bar for NICU performance, and how to measure and support systemwide clinical improvement.

- *"Everyone" means everyone.* As we asserted in Chapter 1, health care improvement is indeed the work of everyone. But we now see that this "everyone" includes not only "each individual" striving for professional excellence but also the collective "everyone," working together in expanding levels of collaboration. The examples in the cases excel not only because they are staffed by talented and committed individuals but also because these individuals bring varied perspectives, skills, and experiences to the common tasks of patient care and system improvement. At the VON collaborative and the VHA PACT, best ideas are shared to the mutual advantage of all participating practices.

Final Reflections

We thus come full circle to the message with which this book began. Practice-based learning and improvement is the work of everyone, which is to say, the work of each of us individually and all of us collectively. We strive together to achieve the common and mutually supportive goals of better patient outcomes, better system performance, and better professional development. The Clinical Value Compass clarifies and coordinates the wide range of outcomes available for improvement work, and the knowledge and skills rehearsed throughout this book (and described in the Clinical Improvement Formula, Chapter 1, Figure 1-3, page 6) empower practitioners to optimize both microsystem and macrosystem performance, even as they support practice-based learning and professional development.[16]

There is enough work to be done, and enough variety of work, to meet the various talents, interests, and personal inclinations of all health care professionals. As we have emphasized repeatedly, improvement work can be practiced independently or collectively, in small informal learning groups or large multidisciplinary collaborations. As we demonstrate in this chapter, this same work can be targeted to settings that are local or regional or even international. Some of us will pursue our improvement mission in the context of solo practice, building simple but meaningful changes into personal work routines. Others will direct attention to ambulatory settings, hospitals or regional networks, or entire health care systems.

Some of us (including authors and editors of this book) will endeavor to develop the educational infrastructure required to advance health professionals' competence in practice-based learning and improvement. We must also commit ourselves to the iterative work of assessment, testing, and reflection, as principles of and experiences in practice-based learning and improvement are introduced early and reinforced throughout undergraduate and graduate health professional education programs.

References

1. Robert Graham Center. The Patient Centered Medical Home: History, Seven Core Features, Evidence and Transformational Change. Nov 2007. Accessed Oct 19, 2012. http://www.graham-center.org/PreBuilt/PCMH.pdf.

2. World Health Organization. Primary Health Care: Report of the International Conference on Primary Health Care[,] Alma-Ata, USSR, 6–12 September 1978. 1978. Accessed Oct 19, 2012. http://whqlibdoc.who.int/publications/9241800011.pdf.

3. Donaldson MS, et al.; Committee on the Future of Primary Care, Institute of Medicine. *Primary Care: America's Health in a New Era.* Washington, DC: National Academy Press, 1996. Accessed Oct 19, 2012. http://www.nap.edu/openbook.php?isbn=0309053994.

4. Spann SJ. Report on financing the new model of family medicine. *Ann Fam Med.* 2004 Dec 2;2 Suppl 3:S1–21.

5. Bodenheimer T, Wagner EH, Grumbach K. Improving primary care for patients with chronic illness: The Chronic Care Model, Part 2. *JAMA.* 2002 Oct 16;288(15):1909–1914.

6. Patient-Centered Primary Care Collaborative. Joint Principles of the Patient-Centered Medical Home. Feb 2007. Accessed Oct 19, 2012. http://www.pcpcc.net/content/joint-principles-patient-centered-medical-home.

7. US Department of Veterans Affairs. VA Centers of Excellence in Primary Care Education. Accessed Oct 19, 2012. http://www.va.gov/oaa/rfp_coe.asp.

8. Vermont Oxford Network: Home page. Accessed Oct 19, 2012. http://www.vtoxford.org.

9. Edwards WH, et al. The effect of prophylactic ointment therapy on nosocomial sepsis rates and skin integrity in infants with birth weights of 501 to 1000 g. *Pediatrics.* 2004 May;113(5):1195–1203.

10. Horbar JD, Soll RF, Edwards WH. The Vermont Oxford Network: A community of practice. *Clin Perinatol.* 2010 Mar;37(1):29–47.

11. National Quality Forum. NQF-Endorsed Standards®. Accessed Oct 19, 2012. http://www.qualityforum.org/Measures_List.aspx.

12. Wirtschafter DD, et al. Nosocomial infection reduction in VLBW infants with a statewide quality-improvement model. *Pediatrics.* 2011 Mar;127(3):419–426.

13. Payne NR, et al. NICU practices and outcomes associated with 9 years of quality improvement collaboratives. *Pediatrics.* 2010 Mar;125(3):437–446.

14. Dunn MS, et al.; Vermont Oxford Network DRM Study Group. Randomized trial comparing 3 approaches to the initial respiratory management of preterm neonates. *Pediatrics.* 2011 Nov;128(5):e1069–1076.

15. American Board of Pediatrics. Addressing the Challenges to Network Sustainability. Presentation at the National Meeting on Collaborative Improvement Networks. Edwards W. Nov 2011. Accessed Oct 19, 2012. https://www.abp.org/abpwebsite/moc/collabimp/William%20Edwards.pdf.

16. Nelson EC, Batalden PB, Godfrey MM, editors. *Quality by Design: A Clinical Microsystems Approach.* San Francisco: Jossey-Bass, 2007.

Afterword

REFLECTING AND IMPROVING IN TIMES LIKE THESE

Paul B. Batalden

Certain phrases come into the lives of health professionals everywhere every day: "Why should I accept your recommendation?" "Your performance numbers are below what we expected." "The first opening in the schedule is much later than I had hoped." "Thank you." "You promised . . ." "This person needs your help."

When science was added to Samaritanism in the eighteenth, nineteenth, and twentieth centuries, it was very disrupting.[1] The familiar routines, the knowledge that needed to be queried and considered, the new syntheses that integrated and combined two disparate knowledge and practice traditions dramatically altered the usual ways and habits of doing professional work. Professionals were challenged in new ways to meet new demands. Eventually people accepted the new paradigm as the most sensible way and became "busy" in this new way of work, like other situations of paradigm shifting.[2] Those faculty and leaders responsible for developing professionals created new pathways of professional development that brought the two traditions together.

In the last few decades, another tradition seems to have been added: social accountability.[3] With it has come universal personal access to information previously reserved for professionals; more information about variation in outcome and process; greater understanding that health care is not the creation of soloist health professionals; keener awareness that the locus for creating health is to be found within the person seeking it; increased recognition that health care resources are always finite and—relative to the need and desire for health—always incomplete; greater need for explicit promise making and more attention

to forgiveness seeking when promises made were not kept. In some ways, similar to the advent of the addition of science to Samaritanism, new knowledge began to emerge, new combinations were needed, new pressures disrupted established ways again—all on top of already full daily calendars.

This book is about changing the work of health professionals living in a three-tradition-grounded reality: Samaritanism, science, and social accountability. It is a book that encourages testing changes. While written so that individuals who read it can benefit, its real impact will come when the functioning small groups of professionals—professionals who are required to work together in today's and tomorrow's health care—read and use it together![4,5]

The simple frames offered in this book invite attention and use of multiple ways of knowing. Each element of the formula denotes a different epistemology[6,7]:

Generalizable science + Particular context →
Measured performance improvement

No particular professional discipline will "own" the future that integrates the three traditions. Whether the health care work creates customized solutions to particular problems, predictably reliable treatments for common problems, or facilitated networks of patients and professionals coproducing services, all will need to understand and integrate the three traditions to create "good value" health care.[8] Changes that are designed to "fit" the simple, complicated, and complex realities they face will be more likely to work and to last.[9,10]

Curiosity and never-ending inquiry into the logic of the "perfectly designed system that produces current levels of performance" will energize the creativity of those involved as they confront the habits, the competing commitments, and the fields of forces at work holding the unchanged present in place.[11–14]

Responding to the integration of these three traditions, each person will know the wisdom that Václav Havel described in his *Letters to Olga**:

It is I who must begin

Once I begin, once I try—
here and now,
right where I am,
not excusing myself
by saying that things
would be easier elsewhere,
without grand speeches and
ostentatious gestures,
but all the more persistently—
to live in harmony
with the voice of Being, as I
understand it within myself
—as soon as I begin that,
I suddenly discover,
to my surprise, that
I am neither the only one,
nor the first,
nor the most important one
to have set out
upon that road.

Whether all is really lost
or not depends entirely on
whether or not I am lost.[15]

Improving health care begins with us as individuals and succeeds when we attract and involve others. Work and use this book together. Now, go for it!

---

* Adapted and arranged in verse form.

References

1. McDermott W. Medicine: The public good and one's own. *Perspect Biol Med.* 1978;21(2):167–187.

2. Kuhn TS. *The Structure of Scientific Revolutions.* Chicago: University of Chicago Press. 1962.

3. Batalden M, Leach D, Batalden P. Better professional development: Competence, mastery, pride and joy. In Batalden P, Foster T, editors: *Sustainably Improving Health Care: Creatively Linking Health Care Outcomes, System Performance and Professional Development.* London: Radcliffe, 2012.

4. Nelson EC, Batalden PB, Godfrey MM, editors. *Quality by Design: A Clinical Microsystems Approach.* San Francisco: Jossey-Bass, 2007.

5. Nelson EC, et al., editors. *Value by Design: Developing Clinical Microsystems to Achieve Organizational Excellence.* San Francisco: Jossey-Bass, 2011.

6. Batalden PB, Davidoff F. What is "quality improvement" and how can it transform healthcare? *Qual Saf Health Care.* 2007 Feb;16(1):2–3.

7. Batalden P, et al. So what? Now what? Exploring, understanding and using the epistemologies that inform the improvement of healthcare. *BMJ Qual Saf.* 2011 Apr;20 Suppl 1:i99–105.

8. Stabel CB, Fjelstad ØD. Configuring value for competitive advantage: On chains, shops, and networks. *Strategic Management Journal.* 1998 May;19(5):413–437.

9. Liu S, Foster T, Batalden P. Simple, complicated, and complex phenomena in health care: Using the triangle to improve reliability and resiliency in health-care systems. In Batalden P, Foster T, editors: *Sustainably Improving Health Care: Creatively Linking Health Care Outcomes, System Performance and Professional Development.* London: Radcliffe, 2012.

10. Glouberman S, Zimmerman B. Complicated and complex systems: What would successful reform of Medicare look like? Discussion paper no. 8. Saskatoon, SK: Commission on the Future of Health Care in Canada, Jul 2002.

11. Patient Safety & Quality in Healthcare. A Quotation with a Life of Its Own. Carr A. Jul–Aug 2008. Accessed Oct 19, 2012. http://www.psqh.com/julaug08/editor.html.

12. Duhigg C. *The Power of Habit: Why We Do What We Do in Life and Business.* New York: Random House, 2012.

13. Kegan R, Lahey LL. *Immunity to Change: How to Overcome It and Unlock the Potential in Yourself and Your Organization.* Boston: Harvard Business School Press, 2009.

14. Lewin K. *Field Theory in Social Science: Selected Theoretical Papers.* New York: Harper, 1951.

15. Havel V. Letter to Olga Havlová, Aug 21, 1982. *Letters to Olga: June 1979–September 1982.* Wilson P, translator. New York: Knopf, 1988, 365–369.

Appendix A

Improving Care: Improvement Worksheets

Eugene C. Nelson, Mary A. Dolansky

Worksheets are helpful tools to guide practice-based learning and improvement. The following worksheets are included in this appendix:

1. Clinical Improvement Worksheet for Teams (Figure A-1, pages 131–134)
2. Clinical Value Compass Worksheet (Figure A-2, pages 135–136)
3. Benchmarking for Best Practices (Figure A-3, pages 137–138)
4. Generic Model for Making and Sustaining Improvements (Figure A-4, pages 139–142)
5. Improvement Project Worksheet (Figure A-5, pages 143–144)

The first four worksheets are intended to be used by individual clinicians for practice-based learning and improvement (or by clinical groups who aim to improve care). The Improvement Project Worksheet (Figure A-5) is a "forest view" of the complete improvement process—a perspective that helps teams understand the full scope of the project. We provide detailed explanation of the steps of the Improvement Project Worksheet (Figure A-5) in this appendix.

The Improvement Project Worksheet

As stated at the top of Side A, the goal is to identify a problem and link current evidence (benchmarking and benchmarks) and system performance (process knowledge). The top section of Side A has spaces to fill in the project title and names of participants in the improvement activity. Group members might wish to designate roles such as leader, facilitator, coach, administrative support, data specialist, or senior leadership champion.

Team Members: Who Should Work on This Improvement?

Consider these guidelines when determining whom to engage in the improvement work:

*   Limit the number of members to eight or fewer for positive group dynamics.
*   Select frontline people who are familiar with key elements of the core process.
*   Reflect diverse areas of expertise and knowledge by including interprofessional staff as well as patients and families.
*   Designate a leader who is credible and responsible for the clinical process.
*   If the group is new to improvement work, consider using an experienced improvement coach or advisor if this expertise is available.

Tips: *Select a set time and day of the week to meet on a regular basis to plan and oversee the first improvement cycle. Structured meeting agendas are recommended.[1] The participants can be a naturally occurring work group (people who normally work together) or a special ad hoc task force specifically assembled—or chartered—to work on a particular clinical area. The participant list should not be finalized until there is a good sense of the patient population that will be targeted for improvement. In practice, it is usually necessary to make a preliminary determination of the selected population and the broad aim (see Step 1, Side A) before selecting the participants.*

Step 1. Problem Identification

What are we trying to accomplish?[2] The team needs to agree on the problem and patient population and identify several criteria to narrow the focus. Potential criteria include procedures or diagnoses that have high volumes, high rates of harm, high costs (including long lengths of stay), high improvement potential per case, intense market competition, high probability of achieving change, importance to stakeholders, and—most important—clinician interest.

Tip: To start the process, consider a target area in which there is both a business need and strong clinician interest. Investment of improvement work in one topic might mean forgoing work on another topic. Reviewing strategy, mission, and data on current performance versus best known performance can help to identify populations for improvement work.

Example: Increased infection rate in the intensive care unit (ICU).

What's the general aim? Start with a broad statement concerning the general, long-term aim for the selected patient population. The general aim statement might touch on multiple aspects of quality, safety, and costs. This general aim statement can be sharpened and made more specific later in the process when preparing for the pilot tests of change.

Tip: The general aim statement can indicate the name of the process, where the process starts and finishes, and what some of the expected benefits of improvement will be.

Example: The process starts when patients are admitted to the ICU and ends when they are discharged. The benefits of improvement are decreased infection rates, lower costs, and increased patient satisfaction.

Step 2. Current Evidence

The next step is for the team to complete a systematic process of searching to identify current evidence of best practices or benchmarking for the problem. Sources can include articles from the literature or other hospital or industry standards. Finding evidence can be facilitated by reading

clinical practice guidelines and looking for *benchmarks,* statistical measures of the results of given practice. The Benchmarking for Best Practices worksheet (Figure A-3) can be used to facilitate this process (for more information, see "Benchmarking for Best Practices: A Planning Worksheet" on pages 60–63 in Chapter 5).

Tip: Calling other hospitals to learn about their processes is an efficient way to learn what others are doing. In addition, the Institute for Healthcare Improvement has a wealth of information, resources, and contacts.[3]

Example: The team addresses finding the evidence and forms three subcommittees. The subcommittees cover the literature, website resources, and contacts with other hospitals.

The team then searches for comparison data on infection rates in the ICU and compares their unit data. The team is also collecting data on the culture of the unit—for example, What other improvement projects has the unit completed? and What is the degree of staff satisfaction with working on the unit?

Step 3. Identification of Current Process— System Performance

What is the process for giving care to this type of patient? Construct a *process diagram*—a flowchart of the care delivery process. Begin by specifying the process boundaries, that is, where the process should start and finish for the selected patient population. For example, the process starts when patients do *X* (for example, enter the emergency department), and the process ends when patients do *Y* (for example, exit the emergency department). The team should construct a first-draft flowchart (graphic mapping) of the delivery process. It is often wise to begin with a simple high-level flowchart (5 to 20 steps) and refine the flowchart over time. Use basic conventions of flowcharting—ovals at the beginning and end of the process, rectangles for main action steps, diamonds for important decision points, and so on.

A *fishbone diagram* (so called because its central "spine" with offshoot branches resembles a fish skeleton; also called a cause-and-effect diagram or an Ishikawa diagram) is useful to identify broad areas for focus. This graphic tool displays the possible causes of a certain effect. The classic fishbone diagram features the categories of materials, methods, equipment, environment, and people. Teams can use this tool to show causes of problems at each step in the process and help identify areas for improvement.

Tips: Make the flowchart big enough for all to view it, and include space for comments. Consider posting it in a place for participants and other staff members to review between meetings. Ask each participant to discuss the improvement work in general and the flowchart specifically with one or two colleagues or patients or family members (who are not participating in this particular improvement) to refine the flowchart and gain better understanding of improvement work rationale and methods. Also make a wall-size illustration (using flipchart pages) of the graphic elements of Side A of the worksheet showing the basic flow of the process to cover the sequence listed in the following section.

As a part of assessing the system, identify the following: Who does what? What equipment is used? What technology is available? What components of the Institute of Medicine aims are involved? This microsystem evaluation will assist the team in understanding what is happening "on the ground" in the specific places where the process unfolds and outcomes are made. Gain an accurate understanding of the physical and structural elements that "front-end load" the work.

Tips: Use direct observation, participant observation, or a combination of the two methods to document important structural features of the actual settings in which the care processes are embedded. How are space and technology used? Are there simple changes that could be made to do the following?

- *Streamline the physical layout.*
- *Clean up messes or untidy places.*
- *Improve the safety of the space.*
- *Have needed equipment in the right place.*
- *Reduce hunting and gathering for supplies.*

- *Feed forward the needed information just in time.*

The team can also assess the culture of the microsystem, including feelings, behaviors, traditions, norms, values, tools, techniques, or outcomes. Are staff members familiar with change and improvement? Have they had prior experiences? Or this their first improvement effort? What is the context? Are staff members ready to make a change? Is there evidence of teamwork? It is important to pay attention to these improvement histories that reflect past attempts to make changes or to do things differently.

Now we move on to Side B of the worksheet. Like Side A, it has a stated goal; the goal of Side B is to define a specific aim, identify measures and interventions, and make a test of change.

Step 4: Specific Aim

Narrowing the general aim helps the team answer the question, "What are we trying to accomplish?" from the Model for Improvement.[2(p. 24)]

Make a more specific aim statement that is in line with the original, general aim statement and that serves as a clear objective for the proposed pilot. In the process of converting the general aim into a more specific aim, sharpen the objective by taking into consideration the relevant aspects of structure, process, and pattern.

Tip: An aim that is specific, measurable, achievable, realistic, and timely (SMART) is necessary to ensure that the goal can be met. If aims are too broad and do not have a realistic time line, success is unlikely. It is important for teams to have success to ensure continual improvement.

Example: Central line–associated bloodstream infections in patients cared for in the ICU will be reduced to one infection per 1,000 line-days within six months.

Step 5 . Measures

This step is reflected in the Model for Improvement with the question, "How will we know that a change is an improvement?"[2(p. 24)]

After narrowing down the aim, select one or two primary outcome measures that can be used to evaluate the success (outcomes and costs) of the pilot test. It is also important to use a countermeasure to detect unwanted side effects; this is called a *balancing measure*. Measurement of process measures helps ensure that the system is performing as planned. Use the Clinical Value Compass and consider clinical outcomes (west), functional and risk status (north), satisfaction against need (east), and then total costs (south). After clarifying the meaning of each brainstormed suggestion, use multivoting to identify the one to three most important measurements in each area.[4]

Tips: *Measures should flow from the specific aim. It is often wise to do the following:*
- *Include fewer rather than more measures to avoid data overload.*
- *Select a few patient descriptors to characterize case mix, a few process measures to indicate how process is changing or staying the same, and a small balanced set of measures of quality and costs.*

See Chapter 4 on measuring outcomes and costs for more detailed instructions on this step. Make a wall-size illustration of the Clinical Value Compass (use flipchart paper), and place the brainstormed ideas and highest-priority results onto the wall directly beside each pertinent compass point. This will build a clear, graphic model for all members of the team to review and refine.

Example: *For each measure, indicate how data will be collected (for example, survey, chart review, direct observation of practice).*

Process Measures: *Identify if and to what degree the change has been implemented, including the following:*
- *Rate of performance of daily review of central line necessity (observe rounds)*
- *Rate of documentation of central line plan in the daily progress note (chart audit)*

Outcome Measures: *Identify if and to what degree the change has resulted in improvement, including the following:*

- *Average length of time central lines are in place (from infection control data)*
- *Central line infection rate (from infection control data)*

Balancing Measures: *Identify if a negative consequence is occurring as a result of the change, such as the following:*
- *Incidence of peripheral IV complications such as infiltrates because central lines are discontinued earlier, resulting in increased use of peripheral IVs (review incident reports)*

Step 6. Identify and Choose Potential Change Ideas

This step is reflected in the Model for Improvement with the question, "What changes can we make that will result in improvement?"[2(p. 24)] Start this step by asking group members to step back for a moment and think about the aim, the desired results (clinical, functional, satisfaction, costs), and the delivery process, patterns, and structural characteristics that they have explored. Then, based on their own ideas and analysis (or based on another person's or expert's ideas or analysis), ask participants to write down (silently and on their own) as many changes as they can think of that might result in better, safer care and lower costs. Ask each member to read one idea, rotating around the group to develop an exhaustive list of change ideas. Clarify these concepts and combine those that are redundant. Use multivoting or another method to help determine the most promising change idea for pilot testing.

Examples: *Each one of the following will be a separate PDSA (Plan–Do–Study–Act) cycle[5]:*
- *Change #1 Hand Hygiene*
- *Change #2 Maximal Barrier Precautions*
- *Change #3 Chlorhexidine Skin Antisepsis for Children 2 Months of Age or Older*
- *Change #4 Optimal Catheter Site Selection*
- *Change #5 Daily Review of Line Necessity*

Step 7: Pilot Test the Change Ideas

The Model for Improvement includes the PDSA tool to assist with pilot testing of interventions.[3]

Plan: *Who? Does What? When? With What Tools and Training?*

Write a brief change protocol that answers these questions. Illustrate the protocol with a simple flowchart.

Tips: A good plan must be executed well to succeed. This means that all involved should know what they are doing and why they are doing it. Writing down the specifics in black and white and illustrating these steps with a flowchart is a good start. Discuss the plan with all those who will be executing it; be prepared to make refinements and changes as needed.

Specify the key questions to be answered by the pilot test, and create a "dummy" version of how data will be displayed to answer these key questions. A dummy data display is a make-believe table or data display that shows exactly how the data will be analyzed and summarized. It often takes the form of a graphic data display showing changes over time using a run chart or control chart or a data table showing results before and after a change is made. Include the operational definitions to be used for each variable in the data collection plan. Whenever possible, build the data collection into the flow of the work; design "self-coding" data collection forms that can be used as care is delivered. Often a pocket-size, preprinted card can be used to gather values on variables that are not routinely or accurately recorded in normal clinical or administrative databases. (Note: Chapter 4, which addresses measuring outcomes and costs, contains more information and a worksheet for operational definitions.)

Do: *What Are We Learning as We Do the Pilot?*

(structure, process, pattern)

Keep a diary of the pilot test. Jot down notes on how the pilot is going, including information on whether all steps are proceeding as planned. Reflect on what is working or failing, and consider the significance of any surprises that might occur.

Tip: Improvement work is full of unanticipated events that might positively or negatively influence the results of the pilot. Also, the results of the pilot will be no better than the care with which the planned change is executed. Observations on the process of change can

prepare the way for making bigger, more powerful changes in the future.

Study: *As We Study and Check What Happened, What Have We Learned?*

Did the original outcomes improve? Analyze the results of the pilot test of change in a way that answers the main question: Did the change lead to the predicted improvement? Were there any unanticipated effects? Were these effects constructive or destructive?

Tip: Consider summarizing the key results graphically and leading off each graph with a question that is answered by the data display. One method of summarizing the results (that links case mix with process changes with outcomes and cost results) is to place before-and-after measures on key points in the process outcome flowchart.

Act: *As We Act to Hold the Gains or Abandon Our Pilot Efforts, What Needs to Be Done?*

If the pilot was successful, and if it was performed on a small scale or a temporary basis, determine what next steps are required to efficiently and effectively build the successful change into daily work routines. Make a plan for mainstreaming the change into daily work and begin to implement it. If the pilot was unsuccessful, analyze the source(s) of the failure. Was this due to a change concept that did not work or a change concept that was not properly implemented? If the former is more likely to be true, then consider going back to the "holding pool" of promising changes and select another for a pilot test.

Tip: Many tests of change fail to produce the desired results. Do not be discouraged; much can be learned from failures. Use this new knowledge to feed into more effective, next-phase change attempts.

After the intervention is determined to work, the next step is to standardize the process to make sure it is sustained. SDSA (Standardize–Do–Study–Act) → How Do We Ensure That Changes Are Standardized and Practiced?

It is common for a change effort to lead to an initial improvement that is lost over time. It is well known that it is easier to make improvements than to make sustained improvements. The question is: How do we hold the gains until further improvements or innovations are made? A good approach to prevent the deterioration of improvement is to recognize the value of monitoring changes between testing (that is, being in a PDSA mode, which involves testing) and sustaining changes (that is, being in an SDSA mode, which involves standardization).

Tip: *Prepare a flowchart to graphically illustrate who does what, when, and in what sequence. This process map can then be used to do the following:*

- *Teach people how to carry out the process in a standard, best-known way*
- *Check actual work routines against the standard routine to promote follow-through and accountability*
- *Serve as the "current process" against which new pilot test processes are compared when switching back over to PDSA mode*

One reason that improvements degrade over time is that people's attention shifts to other matters; there are no reminders nor any way to know that performance is deteriorating. A powerful antidote to this common problem is to use some key measure(s) to monitor performance over time. This is the value of having a valuable, useful, and used "dashboard" or "instrument panel" that offers constant and visual feedback on how things are working.

Tip: *Construct a "data wall" to serve as a "dashboard" that monitors key performance indicators. Review and discuss the dashboard metrics on a regular basis with all the members of the microsystem who are engaged in the process and who therefore contribute to the outcomes. A visually rich information environment is a powerful trigger to action. If dashboard measures are staying in the "right zone," this suggests that the new process is continuing to function correctly. If metrics decline (rapidly or gradually) or if they vary widely, "upstream" or underlying conditions might have changed, in which case further improvements must be considered. Alternatively, conditions have remained stable, and the initial improvement is still viable, but retraining of staff is required.*

References

1. Scholtes PR, Joiner BL, Streibel BJ. *The Team Handbook,* 3rd ed. Madison, WI: Oriel, 2003.
2. Langley GJ, et al. *The Improvement Guide: A Practical Approach to Enhancing Organizational Performance,* 2nd ed. San Francisco: Jossey-Bass, 2009.
3. Institute for Healthcare Improvement. Home Page. Accessed Oct 19, 2012. http://www.IHI.org.
4. Nelson EC, et al. Good measurement for good improvement work. *Qual Manag Health Care.* 2004 Jan–Mar;13(1):1–16.
5. Institute for Healthcare Improvement. Implement the IHI Central Line Bundle. (Updated Aug 2, 2011.) Accessed Oct 19, 2012. http://www.ihi.org/knowledge/Pages/Changes/ImplementtheCentralLineBundle.aspx.

Figure A-1. Clinical Improvement Worksheet for Teams, Side A

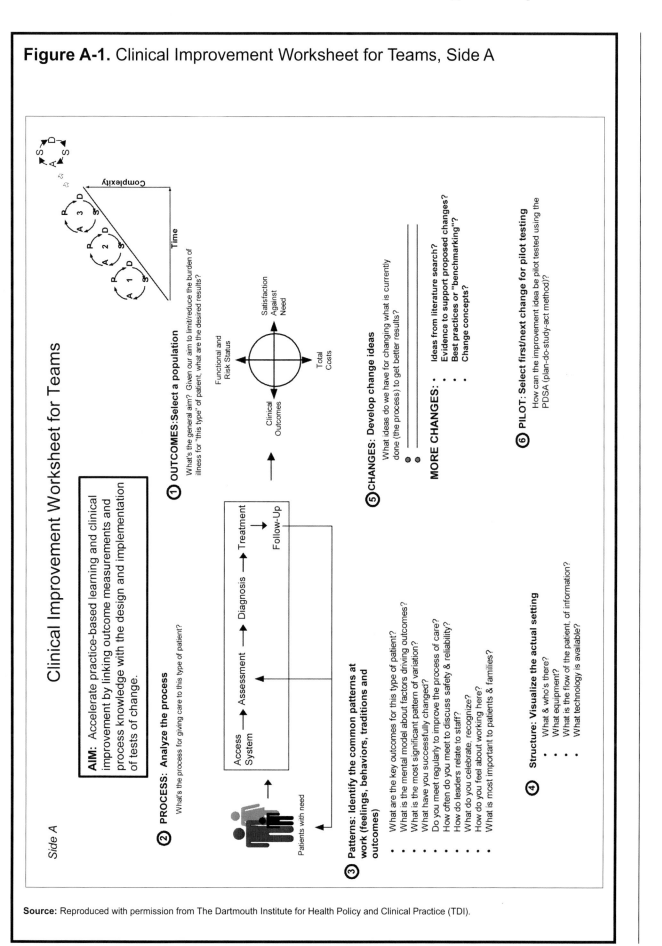

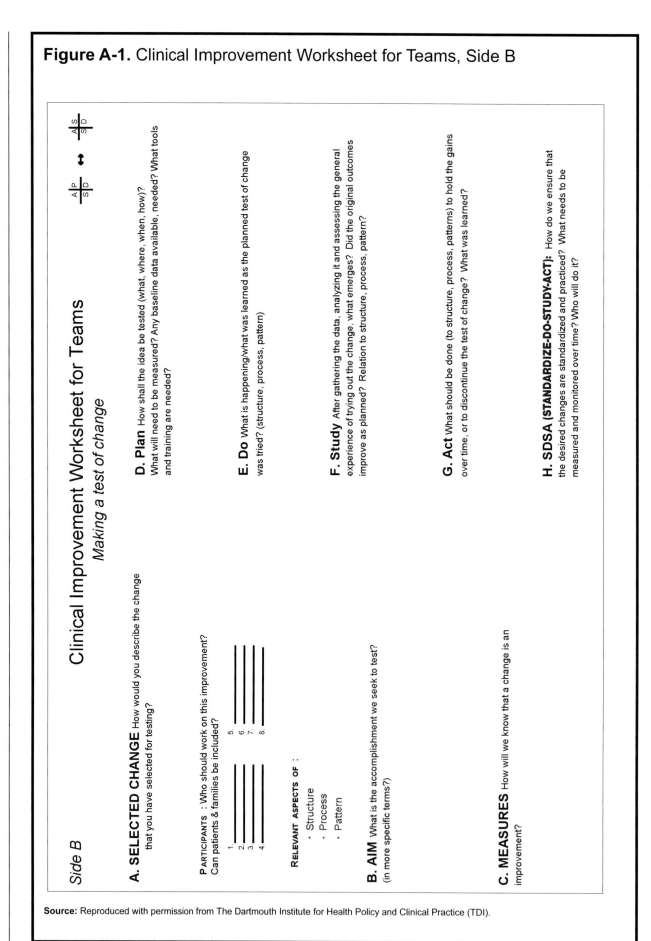

Figure A-1. Clinical Improvement Worksheet for Teams, Side B

Source: Reproduced with permission from The Dartmouth Institute for Health Policy and Clinical Practice (TDI).

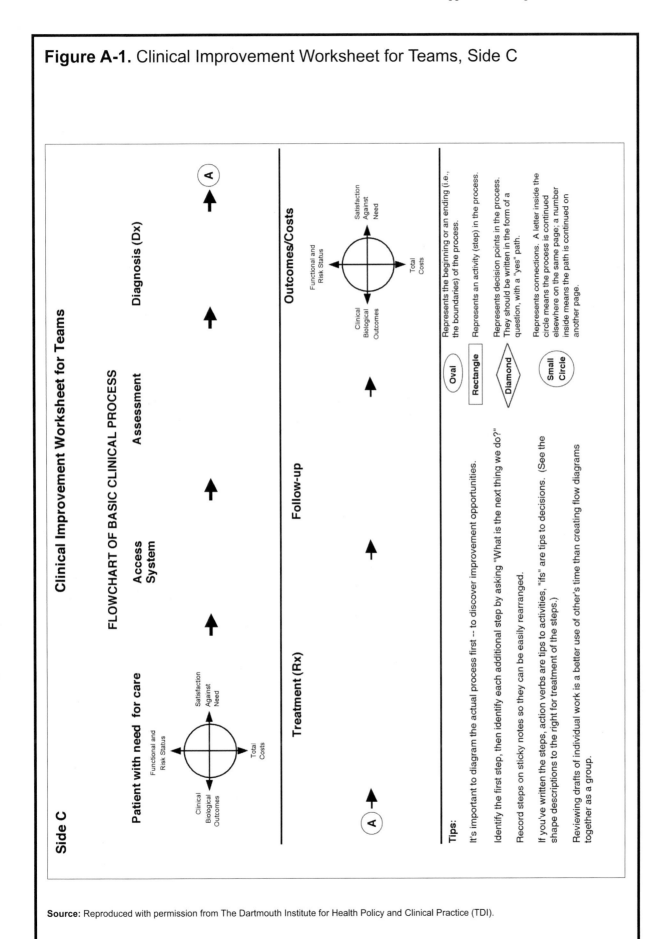

Figure A-1. Clinical Improvement Worksheet for Teams, Side C

Figure A-1. Clinical Improvement Worksheet for Teams, Side D

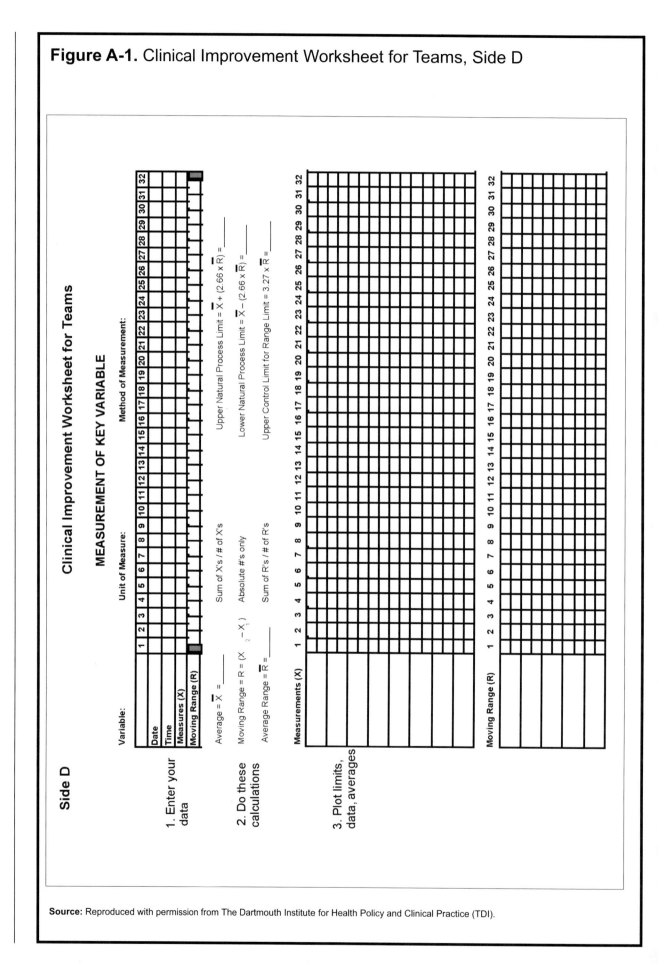

Source: Reproduced with permission from The Dartmouth Institute for Health Policy and Clinical Practice (TDI).

Figure A-2. Clinical Value Compass Worksheet, Side A

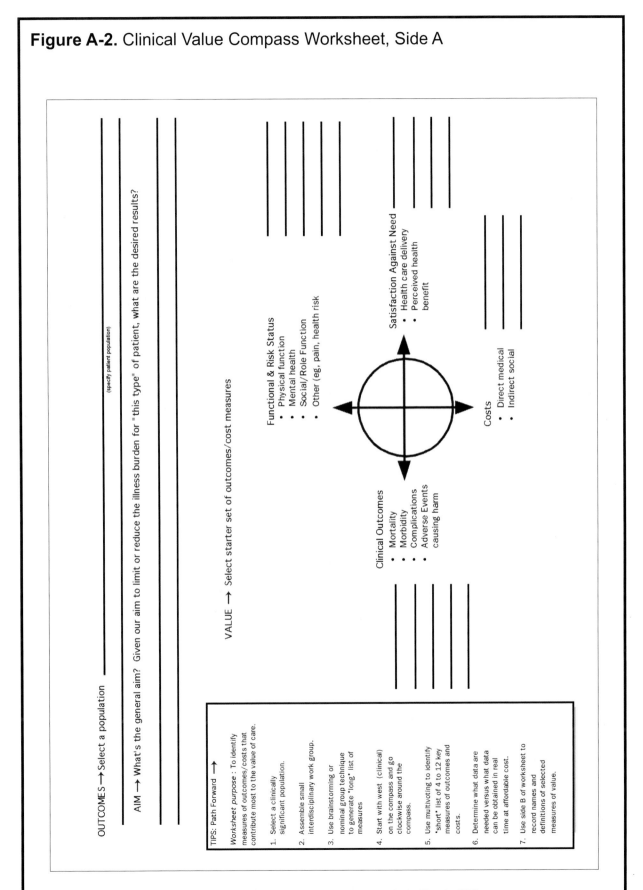

OUTCOMES → Select a population _____
(specify patient population)

AIM → What's the general aim? Given our aim to limit or reduce the illness burden for "this type" of patient, what are the desired results?

VALUE → Select starter set of outcomes/cost measures

Functional & Risk Status
• Physical function
• Mental health
• Social/Role Function
• Other (eg, pain, health risk

Satisfaction Against Need
• Health care delivery
• Perceived health benefit

Costs
• Direct medical
• Indirect social

Clinical Outcomes
• Mortality
• Morbidity
• Complications
• Adverse Events causing harm

TIPS: Path Forward ↑

Worksheet purpose : To identify measures of outcomes/costs that contribute most to the value of care.

1. Select a clinically significant population.

2. Assemble small interdisciplinary work group.

3. Use brainstorming or nominal group technique to generate "long" list of measures

4. Start with west (clinical) on the compass and go clockwise around the compass.

5. Use multivoting to identify "short" list of 4 to 12 key measures of outcomes and costs.

6. Determine what data are needed versus what data can be obtained in real time at affordable cost.

7. Use side B of worksheet to record names and definitions of selected measures of value.

Figure A-2. Clinical Value Compass Worksheet, Side B

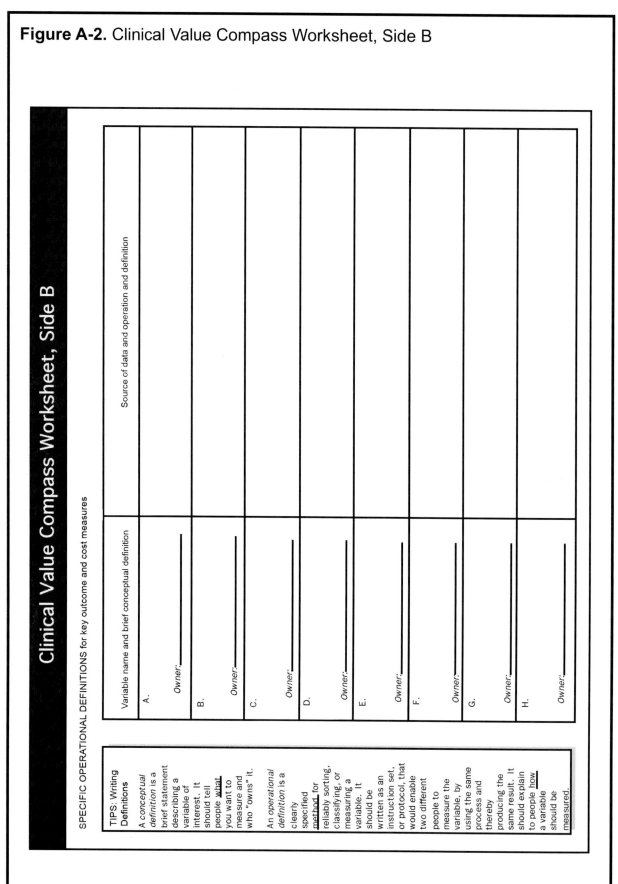

Figure A-3. Benchmarking for Best Practices, Side A

Aim: Develop ideas about best practices.

1. Identify measures.

Using the Clinical Value Compass as a guide, reach a consensus on 2 or 3 statistical measures, or benchmarks, that will be the focus of the external scan. Consider the availability of valid comparative data and variability of performance across facilities. (An appropriate benchmark enables measurement and comparison across systems.)

Functional Health Status

Clinical Outcomes

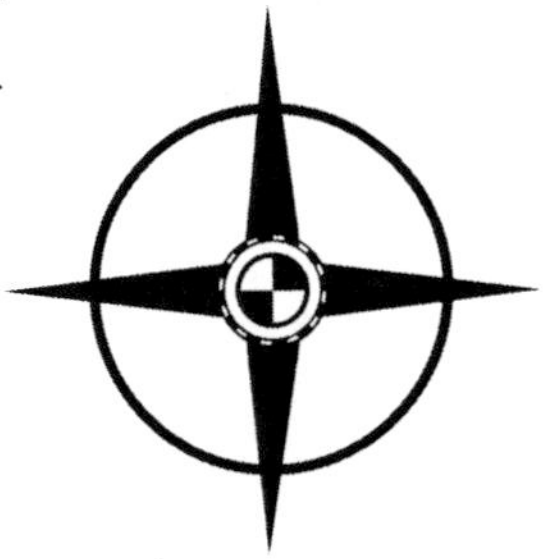

Satisfaction Against Need

Total Costs

2. Determine resources needed to find the best of the best.

Given our desire to limit or reduce the illness burden (cost, resource use, excess morbidity, mortality) for our patients, think about the information needed for finding the best of the best.

The best data to use?
Internal?

External?

The best people to ask?
In-house?

Out-of-house?

The best literature?

Source: Reproduced with permission from The Dartmouth Institute for Health Policy and Clinical Practice (TDI).

Figure A-3. Benchmarking for Best Practices, Side B

3. **Design data-collection method and gather data.**
   Who will collect the data? How will the data be analyzed? Who will review the literature?

   Task: Person completing: Date to be completed:

   _____

   _____

   _____

   _____

   _____

   _____

   _____

4. **Measure best against own performance to determine gap.**
   Based on the measures identified in step 1, and the results of an internal and external scan of the data, how does our performance compare to the best of the best?

   Benchmark: _____

   Our results   _____
   Average   _____
   "Best"   _____

   Benchmark: _____

   Our results   _____
   Average   _____
   "Best"   _____

Summary Data	
Number of cases:	_____
Total revenue:	_____
Revenue rank:	_____

   Benchmark: _____

   Our results   _____
   Average   _____
   "Best"   _____

   Benchmark: _____

   Our results   _____
   Average   _____
   "Best"   _____

   Functional Health Status

   Clinical Outcomes — **Satisfaction Against Need**

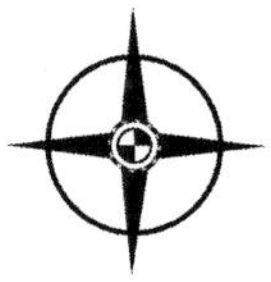

   Total Costs

   Compared to what we found, how good is our quality and value?

   Benchmark: _____

   Our results   _____
   Average   _____
   "Best"   _____

   Benchmark: _____

   Our results   _____
   Average   _____
   "Best"   _____

5. **Identify the best practices that produce best-in-class results.**

Source: Reproduced with permission from The Dartmouth Institute for Health Policy and Clinical Practice (TDI).

Figure A-4. Generic Model for Making and Sustaining Improvements:
PDSA ↔ SDSA Worksheet, Side A

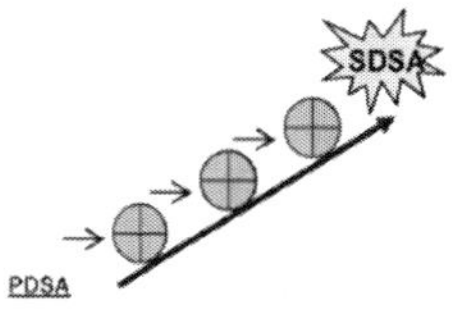

PDSA ↔ SDSA Worksheet

Name of Group: _____   Start Date: _____

TEAM MEMBERS

1. Leader: _____   5. _____
2. Facilitator: _____   6. _____
3. _____   7. _____
4. _____   8. _____

Coach: _____   Meeting Day/Time: _____

Data Support: _____   Place: _____

1. *Aim* ➡ What are we trying to accomplish?

2. *Measures* ➡ How will we know that a change is an improvement?

3. *Current Process* ➡ What is the process for giving care to this type of patient?

Note: Questions 1, 2, and 3 are bigger picture (30,000 feet type) questions.
     Questions 4–8 are very specific, ground-level questions.
This worksheet can be used to plan and keep track of improvement efforts.

Figure A-4. Generic Model for Making and Sustaining Improvements: PDSA ↔ SDSA Worksheet, Side B

Plan ➤ How shall we PLAN the pilot? Who does what and when? With what tools or training?
  • Baseline data to be collected? How will we know if a change is an improvement?

Tasks to be completed to run test of change	Who	When	Tools/Training Needed	Measures

Do ➤ What are we learning as we *DO* the pilot? What happened when we ran the test? Any problems encountered? Any surprises?

Study ➤ As we *STUDY* what happened, what have we learned? What do the measures show?

Act ➤ As we *ACT* to hold the gains or abandon our pilot efforts, what needs to be done? Will we modify the change? Make PLAN for the next cycle of change.

Standardize ➤ Once you have determined this PDSA result to be the current "best practice" take action to Standardize-Do-Study-Act (SDSA). You will create the conditions to ensure this "best practice" in daily activities until a NEW change is identified and then the SDSA moves back to the PDSA cycle to test the idea to then standardize again.

Source: Reproduced with permission from The Dartmouth Institute for Health Policy and Clinical Practice (TDI).

Figure A-4. Generic Model for Making and Sustaining Improvements: PDSA ↔ SDSA Worksheet, Side C

Tradeoffs ➔ What are we NOT going to do anymore to support this new habit?

What has helped us in the past to change behavior and helped us do the "right thing?"

What type of environment has supported standardization?

How do we design the new "best practice" to be the default step in the process?

Consider professional behaviors, attitudes, values, and assumptions when designing how to embed this new "best practice."

Measures ➔ How will we know that this process continues to be an improvement?

What measures will inform us if "standardization" is in practice?

How will we know if "old behaviors" have appeared again?

How will we measure? How often? Who?

This worksheet can be used to plan-standardize and keep track of improvement efforts.

Source: Reproduced with permission from The Dartmouth Institute for Health Policy and Clinical Practice (TDI).

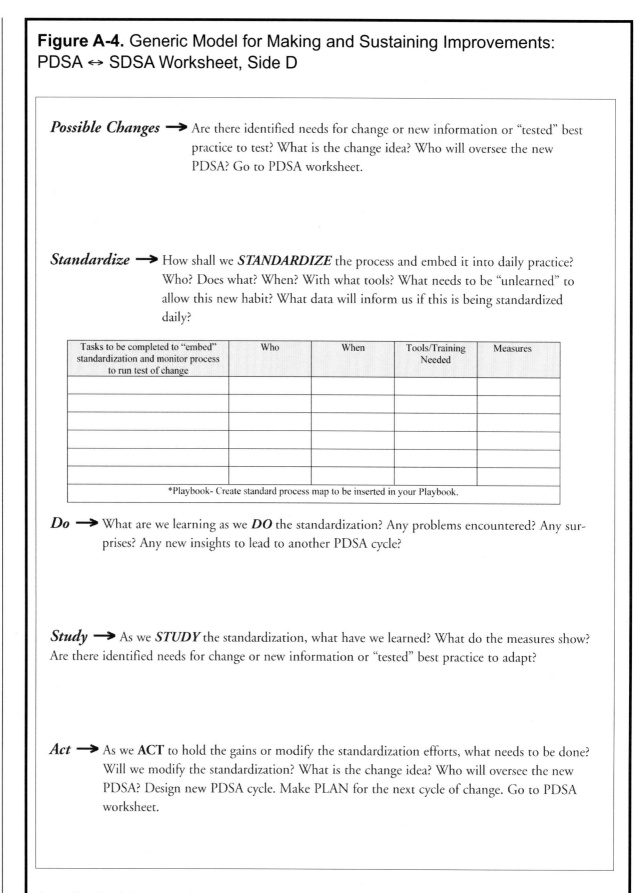

Figure A-4. Generic Model for Making and Sustaining Improvements: PDSA ↔ SDSA Worksheet, Side D

Possible Changes → Are there identified needs for change or new information or "tested" best practice to test? What is the change idea? Who will oversee the new PDSA? Go to PDSA worksheet.

Standardize → How shall we ***STANDARDIZE*** the process and embed it into daily practice? Who? Does what? When? With what tools? What needs to be "unlearned" to allow this new habit? What data will inform us if this is being standardized daily?

Tasks to be completed to "embed" standardization and monitor process to run test of change	Who	When	Tools/Training Needed	Measures
*Playbook- Create standard process map to be inserted in your Playbook.				

Do → What are we learning as we ***DO*** the standardization? Any problems encountered? Any surprises? Any new insights to lead to another PDSA cycle?

Study → As we ***STUDY*** the standardization, what have we learned? What do the measures show? Are there identified needs for change or new information or "tested" best practice to adapt?

Act → As we ***ACT*** to hold the gains or modify the standardization efforts, what needs to be done? Will we modify the standardization? What is the change idea? Who will oversee the new PDSA? Design new PDSA cycle. Make PLAN for the next cycle of change. Go to PDSA worksheet.

Source: Reproduced with permission from The Dartmouth Institute for Health Policy and Clinical Practice (TDI).

Figure A-5. Improvement Project Overview Worksheet, Side A

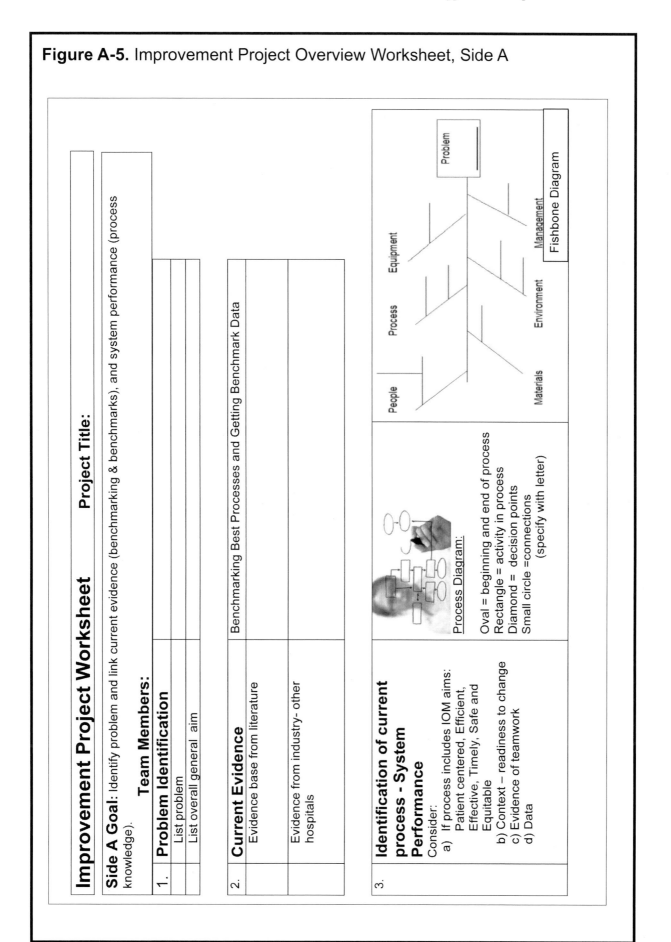

Improvement Project Worksheet   **Project Title:**

Side A Goal: Identify problem and link current evidence (benchmarking & benchmarks), and system performance (process knowledge).

Team Members:

1.	**Problem Identification**
	List problem
	List overall general aim

2.	**Current Evidence**	Benchmarking Best Processes and Getting Benchmark Data
	Evidence base from literature	
	Evidence from industry- other hospitals	

3.	**Identification of current process - System Performance** Consider: a) If process includes IOM aims: Patient centered, Efficient, Effective, Timely, Safe and Equitable b) Context – readiness to change c) Evidence of teamwork d) Data	Process Diagram: Oval = beginning and end of process Rectangle = activity in process Diamond = decision points Small circle =connections (specify with letter)	People Process Equipment Materials Environment Management Problem Fishbone Diagram

Figure A-5. Improvement Project Overview Worksheet, Side B

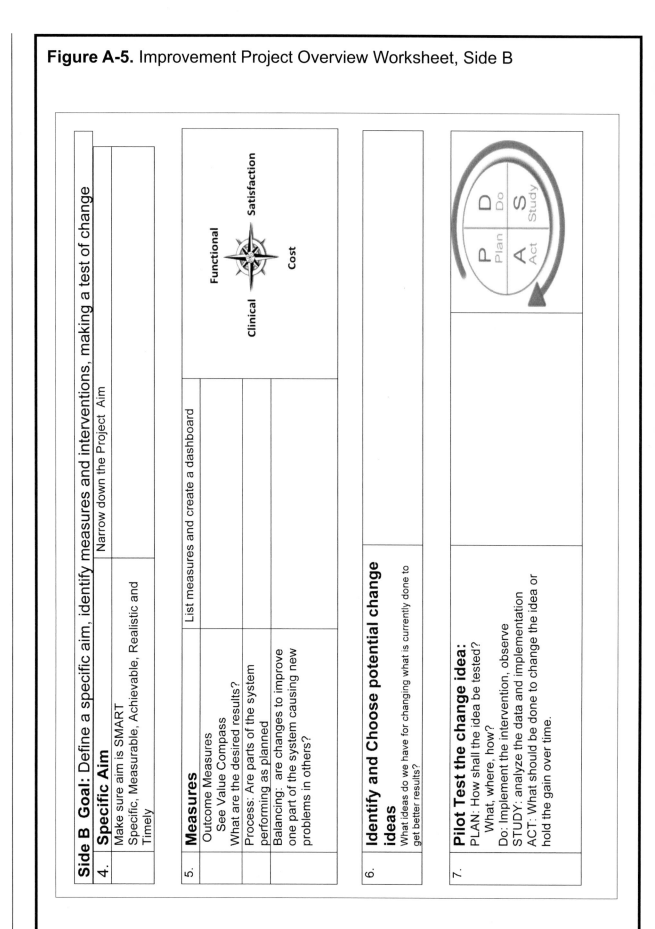

Side B Goal: Define a specific aim, identify measures and interventions, making a test of change

4.	Specific Aim	Narrow down the Project Aim
	Make sure aim is SMART Specific, Measurable, Achievable, Realistic and Timely	

5.	Measures	List measures and create a dashboard
	Outcome Measures See Value Compass What are the desired results?	
	Process: Are parts of the system performing as planned	
	Balancing: are changes to improve one part of the system causing new problems in others?	

6.	Identify and Choose potential change ideas
	What ideas do we have for changing what is currently done to get better results?

7.	Pilot Test the change idea:
	PLAN: How shall the idea be tested? What, where, how? Do: Implement the intervention, observe STUDY: analyze the data and implementation ACT: What should be done to change the idea or hold the gain over time.

Appendix B

Observational and Interviewing Worksheets

Eugene C. Nelson, Marjorie M. Godfrey

The ultimate aim of improvement in health care is to find better and better ways to meet the patient's and family's needs and thereby to decrease the burden of illness and increase the level of wellness experienced by the patient and family.

The focus of this appendix is to provide information on observations and interviews. These tools can be used to gain insight into the way things really work, which drives outcomes, and into the perceptions of patients and families about the quality of the care that they receive, which drives satisfaction and loyalty.[1]

No methods for understanding what to do to improve care in a particular health care setting are more powerful than using observations and interviews. There are various ways to conduct observations and interviews, such as the following:

- **Participant observation:** taking part in care delivery and reflecting on what is seen, heard, and felt
- **Direct observation:** looking in on actual (or simulated) care being delivered and analyzing the process to detect inefficiency, unreliability, and unsafe practices and working conditions
- **Individual interviews:** conducting a focused conversation with individual patients and individual family members to gain deep insight into how they perceive their health and their experiences in receiving health care

Participant Observation: A Way to Reveal Patients' Perceptions of Their Experience

One powerful observational technique is to set up situations that enable one to experience (see, hear, talk, feel) patients' health care journeys as they do; that is, to "walk in their shoes." Using the worksheet Through the Eyes of Your Patients (Figure B-1, page 148) provides an opportunity to see the journey—the visit to the office, the visit to the emergency department, the time spent in an inpatient care unit, the home visit by a visiting nurse—from the patient and family perspective. This technique uses role playing to simulate the experiences of being a patient (or a family member of a patient) with a certain health condition receiving care in a specific context. Through the Eyes of Your Patients offers simple guidance for using this powerful observational method. It is particularly useful to gain a better understanding of the patient's and family's subjective impressions (their perceptions) about how they are being treated, which shapes people's evaluation of the quality of the care that they receive.

Direct Observation: A Way to Uncover Waste, Rework, Unreliability, and Threats to Safety and Reliability

Another powerful observational technique used extensively in many of the most successful and improvement-oriented organizations in the world (such as Toyota) is direct observation of the "real work." Improvement often starts with careful observation and reflection on how things are done in the real world under normal operating conditions. Does the process include unnecessary effort, rework, extra steps, work-arounds, unreliable features, potential safety threats, or waste of any kind (motion, resources, and so on)? These observations can generate a deep, accurate understanding of the processes and can be used to identify process imperfections associated with waste, rework, unreliability, and threats to safety. The Clinical Microsystem Observation Worksheet (Figure B-2, page 149) provides a method for documenting process flows—the way things work—on the basis of the observed patient experience in a specific clinical context.

For a more elaborate approach to work flow observation, a useful technique is value stream mapping, a sophisticated, detailed process analysis method that includes both the sequence of actions and the flow of information that is associated with the actions.[2,3]

Individual Interviews: A Way to Learn About Perceptions on Being Cared For and Receiving Care

Individual interviews offer another powerful yet flexible method for gaining knowledge about the patient's and family's perceptions of their experiences in health care and about their interactions with physicians, nurses, and other staff. Holding a special, private conversation with a patient—or with a family member who is part of that patient's support system—can produce a bounty of stories, insights, and impressions that are perceived as important aspects of the process of caring, the nature of the relationships, and the perceived benefits stemming from the health care received. The Clinical Microsystem Interview Worksheet (Figure B-3, pages 150–152) provides a path for planning and conducting individual interviews.

Another well-known approach for gaining qualitative information is to use focus group interviewing.[4,5] This too is a flexible yet powerful method but requires greater expertise and more detailed planning and logistics than individual, in-depth interviews.

Observing the "Real Work" of Clinical Care

The plastic surgery section at Dartmouth-Hitchcock Medical Center has been actively engaged in efforts to improve local care. Team members have worked toward the interdependent goals of optimizing patient outcomes and (through elimination of waste and rework in the process of care) creating a more joyful work experience for clinicians and staff members themselves. The use of observation techniques has been extremely beneficial to the improvement effort.

In the endoscopic surgical treatment of carpal tunnel syndrome, for example, video recording the entire procedure has led to significant improvements in perioperative surgical care processes. Review of the recordings, which include all interventions from initial setup to final cleanup, has enabled team members to see many opportunities for improvement that were previously hidden, including elimination of waste and reduction in unnecessary variation.

The advantage of video recording is that all members of a practice team can visualize current processes as they occur in the real world. This visualization promotes recognition of specific improvement opportunities and facilitates buy-in of all participants, who can then work together to modify activities and eliminate waste. For the plastic surgery team, the video recording highlighted variation between two registered nurses who assisted the surgeon on different days, resulting in highly varied processes. When the lead improvement team reviewed the recording, it was able to create process maps and highlight best practices. The nurses were then empowered to standardize the process, resulting in benefit to both patients and staff.

This new standardization enabled the surgeon to increase her productivity from three or four carpal tunnel procedures to six to eight procedures per session. At the same time, specific responsibilities in the care process could be matched more effectively to specific team members on the basis of education, training, and licensure, thereby freeing time for the surgeon and the nurse to engage in other appropriate activities within the practice. Finally, the group was able to build standard carpal tunnel kits and to decrease the number of surgical packs from six to two; procedures for setup and cleanup were standardized as well. Because of these and other new efficiencies, the same practice has more recently been able to run two procedure rooms at the same time, greatly enhancing productivity with no reduction in quality of care.

References

1. Lee F. *If Disney Ran Your Hospital: 9½ Things You Would Do Differently.* Bozeman, MT: Second River Healthcare, 2004.
2. George ML, et al. *The Lean Six Sigma Pocket Toolbook.* New York: McGraw-Hill, 2005.
3. Rother M, Shook H. *Learning to See: Value-Stream Mapping to Create Value and Eliminate Muda,* ver. 1.1. Cambridge, MA: Lean Enterprise Institute, 1998.
4. Morgan DL, Krueger RA, editors. *The Focus Group Kit,* vols. 1–6. Thousand Oaks, CA: Sage, 1997.
5. Stewart DW, Shamdasani PN. *Focus Groups: Theory and Practice.* Applied Social Research Methods Series, vol. 20. Newbury Park, CA: Sage, 1990.

Figure B-1. Through the Eyes of Your Patients: A Guide to Conducting a Patient-Experience Simulation of Care

Patients

Aim: Gain insight into how your patients experience the process of interacting with clinical services. One simple way to understand both patient flow and patient perceptions of receiving care is to experience the care through the eyes of a patient. Members of your staff can do a simulated care experience by "walking through" the care experience using role playing to simulate care delivery. Try to make this experience as real as possible; this form can be used to document the experience. You can also capture the patient experience by making an audio or videotape.

Through the Eyes of Your Patients

Tips for making the "walk through" most productive:

1. Determine with your staff where the starting point and ending points should be, taking into consideration appointment making or entering the clinical system, admissions, the actual office visit or clinical care process, follow-up, and other issues you may suspect are problems.
2. Two members of the staff should do the walk through together if possible, with each playing a role: patient and partner/family member.
3. Set aside a reasonable amount of time to experience the patient journey. Consider the usual amount of time patients spend in your clinic or in your clinical unit.

4. Make it real. Have a real appointment with a real clinician or a real visit to an emergency department, or other typical process of being admitted or discharged from an inpatient unit. Include time with lab tests, and arranging for reports to be delivered. Sit where the patient sits, lie where the patient lies. Wear what the patient wears. Make a realistic paper trail including chart, lab reports, discharge planning, and payment arrangements.
5. During the walk-through note both positive and negative experiences, as well as any surprises. What was frustrating? What was gratifying? What was confusing? Again, an audio or video tape can be helpful.
6. Debrief your staff on what you did and what you learned.

Date: _____   Staff Members: _____

Walk Through Begins When: _____   Ends When: _____

Positives	Negatives	Surprises	Frustrating/Confusing	Gratifying

Figure B-2. Clinical Microsystem Observation Worksheet

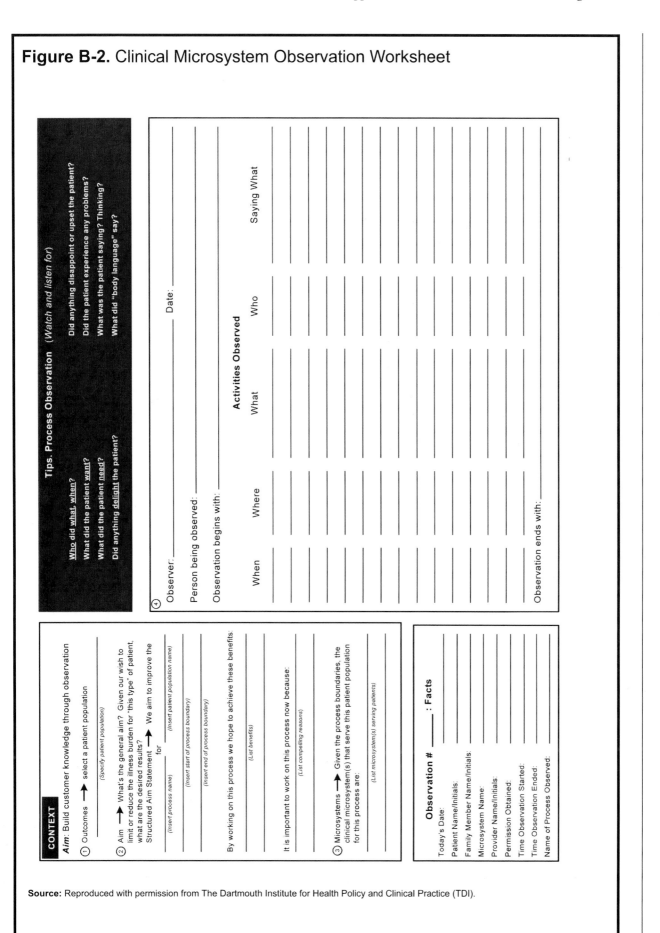

Figure B-3. Clinical Microsystem Interview Worksheet

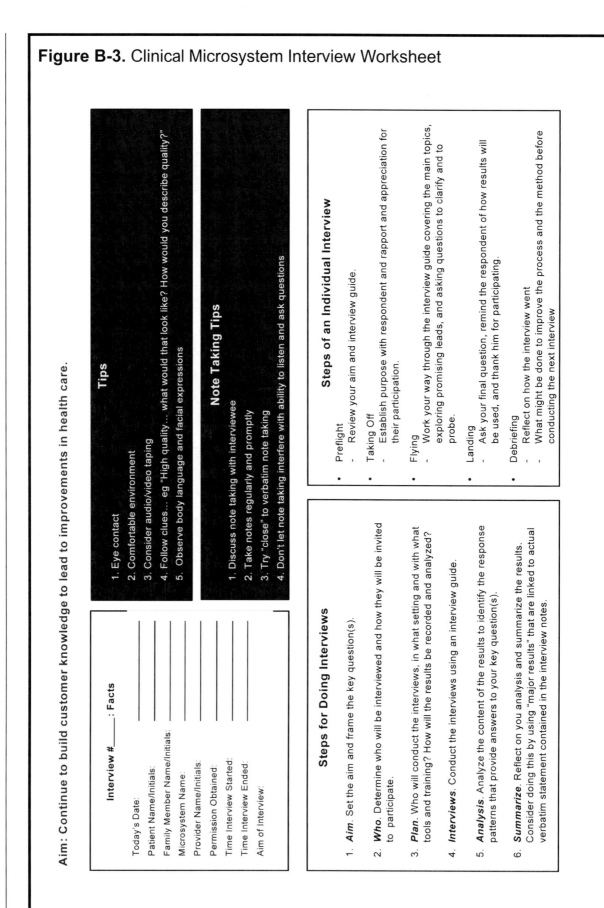

Aim: Continue to build customer knowledge to lead to improvements in health care.

Interview # _____ : Facts

Today's Date:
Patient Name/Initials:
Family Member Name/Initials:
Microsystem Name:
Provider Name/Initials:
Permission Obtained:
Time Interview Started:
Time Interview Ended:
Aim of Interview:

Tips

1. Eye contact
2. Comfortable environment
3. Consider audio/video taping
4. Follow clues… eg "High quality… what would that look like? How would you describe quality?"
5. Observe body language and facial expressions

Note Taking Tips

1. Discuss note taking with interviewee
2. Take notes regularly and promptly
3. Try "close" to verbatim note taking
4. Don't let note taking interfere with ability to listen and ask questions

Steps of an Individual Interview

• Preflight
  - Review your aim and interview guide.

• Taking Off
  - Establish purpose with respondent and rapport and appreciation for their participation.

• Flying
  - Work your way through the interview guide covering the main topics, exploring promising leads, and asking questions to clarify and to probe.

• Landing
  - Ask your final question, remind the respondent of how results will be used, and thank him for participating.

• Debriefing
  - Reflect on how the interview went
  - What might be done to improve the process and the method before conducting the next interview

Steps for Doing Interviews

1. **Aim.** Set the aim and frame the key question(s).

2. **Who.** Determine who will be interviewed and how they will be invited to participate.

3. **Plan.** Who will conduct the interviews, in what setting and with what tools and training? How will the results be recorded and analyzed?

4. **Interviews.** Conduct the interviews using an interview guide.

5. **Analysis.** Analyze the content of the results to identify the response patterns that provide answers to your key question(s).

6. **Summarize.** Reflect on you analysis and summarize the results. Consider doing this by using "major results" that are linked to actual verbatim statement contained in the interview notes.

continued on next page

Figure B-3. Clinical Microsystem Interview Worksheet, *continued*

Gaining Customer Knowledge
Clinical Microsystem Interview Worksheet

Interview Guide Template

⑤

Preflight

- Interview who, where, under what auspices, with what guide, for what purpose

Taking Off

- Introduce self, purpose of interview, how information is to be used, assure confidentiality, ask any questions and ask permission to proceed with the interview.
- First question . . . Write an open-ended question that invites the respondent to tell his/her "story" re: topic of interest . . .

My first question is: _____

Flying

- Frame several "core" questions to achieve your aim and answer key questions.

1. _____
2. _____
3. _____
4. _____
5. _____

Landing

- Last question . . . Write summative last question. . . .

My last question is: _____

- Thank respondent and say goodbye.

Debriefing

- If taking notes . . . Review notes and add to them to make as complete a record as possible
- Consider what new is learned by this interview
- Consider refinements to interview guide based on what was learned

continued on next page

Figure B-3. Clinical Microsystem Interview Worksheet, *continued*

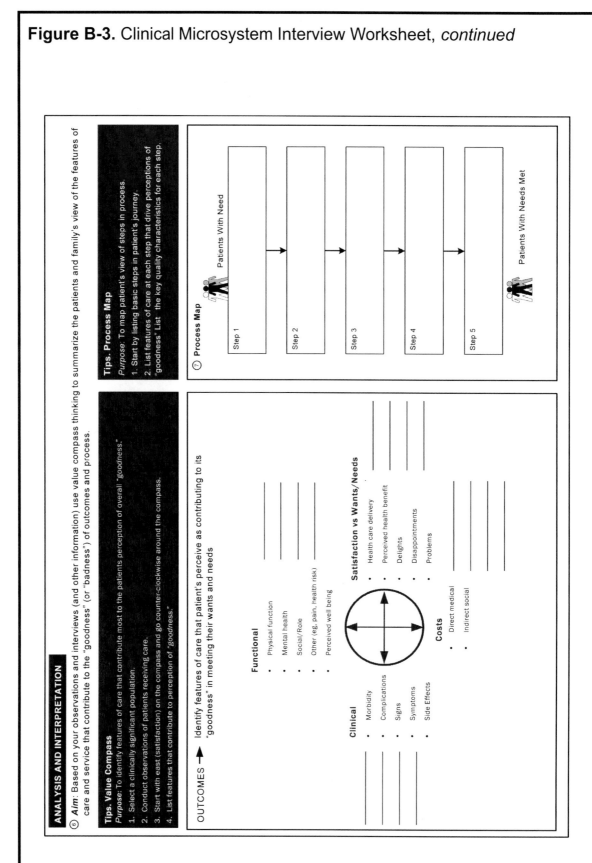

Source: Reproduced with permission from The Dartmouth Institute for Health Policy and Clinical Practice (TDI).

Appendix C

MEASURES OF QUALITY AND VALUE

Mary A. Dolansky, Carlos A. Estrada

Methods for measuring quality and value are advancing rapidly, and their use is proliferating. Policy makers, researchers, practitioners, payers, and patients are increasingly vocal in their demand for better measures of quality and costs. Table C-1, below, contains a list of organizations and useful resources to consider when examining patient-reported measures of quality; the list is by no means exhaustive.

Table C-1. Organizations and Resources

Organization	Description	Website
Agency for Healthcare Research and Quality Consumer Assessment of Healthcare Providers and Systems (CAHPS)	The acronym CAHPS refers to a comprehensive and evolving set of surveys that ask consumers and patients to evaluate the interpersonal aspects of health care. CAHPS surveys determine those aspects of care for which consumers and patients are the best and/or only source of information, as well as those that consumers and patients have identified as being important.	http://cahps.ahrq.gov
Dartmouth Atlas of Health Care	The site provides an interactive system for benchmarking to compare the experience in areas or hospitals of your choice to the national average, state average, or the rate in other areas or hospitals.	http://www.dartmouthatlas.org/tools/benchmarking.aspx
Institute for Healthcare Improvement's Whole System Measures (2007)	This white paper describes and promotes the use of a system of metrics, called the Whole System Measures, to measure the overall quality of a health system and to align improvement work across a hospital, group practice, or large health care system.	http://www.ihi.org/knowledge/Pages/IHIWhitePapers/WholeSystemMeasuresWhitePaper.aspx
Institute of Medicine's Performance Measurement: Accelerating Improvement (2005)	This document provides a framework and implementation strategy for translating public and professional concerns about performance and accountability into measures of health care quality.	http://www7.nationalacademies.org/ocga/briefings/Performance_Measurement.asp
Leapfrog Group	The Leapfrog Group aims to (1) inform Americans about their hospital safety and quality, (2) promote full public disclosure of hospital performance information, and (3) help employers provide the best health care benefits to their employees. Performance measures are listed on the reports.	http://leapfroggroup.org

continued on next page

Table C-1. Organizations and Resources, *continued*

Organization	Description	Website
The Joint Commission	The mission of The Joint Commission is to continuously improve health care for the public, in collaboration with other stakeholders, by evaluating health care organizations and inspiring them to excel in providing safe and effective care of the highest quality and value. The Joint Commission website contains performance measures, accountability measures, and core measure sets.	http://www.jointcommission.org/performance_measurement.aspx
Joint Commission Quality Check®	Quality Check® is the most comprehensive listing of health care organizations available today. Joint Commission accreditation/certification is recognized nationwide as a symbol of quality and safety that reflects an organization's commitment to meeting certain performance standards. In the Quality Report, data on patient satisfaction (Survey of Patients' Hospital Experiences) may be obtained.	http://www.qualitycheck.org
National Database of Nursing Quality Indicators (NDNQI)	The NDNQI is a proprietary database of the American Nurses Association. The database collects and evaluates unit-specific nurse-sensitive data from hospitals in the United States.	https://www.nursingquality.org
National Quality Forum Measure Applications Partnership (MAP)	MAP is a public-private partnership that reviews performance measures for potential use in federal public reporting and performance-based payment programs. It aligns public programs with measures being used in the private sector. MAP is the first group of its kind to provide upstream, prerule-making input to the federal government on the selection of quality measures.	http://www.qualityforum.org/map/
National Quality Measures Clearinghouse (NQMC)	The NQMC is a public resource for evidenced-based quality measures and measure sets.	http://www.qualitymeasures.ahrq.gov
Patient Reported Outcomes Measurement Information System (PROMIS)	Funded by the National Institutes of Health, PROMIS is a system of reliable, valid, flexible, precise, and responsive assessment tools measuring patient-reported health status.	http://www.nihpromis.org
Physician Consortium for Performance Improvement (PCPI)	The American Medical Association convened the PCPI in the early 2000s with the goal of enhancing quality and patient safety and fostering accountability. The PCPI continues to lead efforts in developing, testing, and implementing evidence-based performance measures.	http://www.ama-assn.org/ama/pub/physician-resources/physician-consortium-performance-improvement.page

Appendix D

COLLECTING DATA: PRINCIPLES AND GUIDELINES FOR SUCCESS

Eugene C. Nelson

Principles for Using Data in Clinical Practice for Learning and Improvement

1. Keep Measurement Simple: Think Big and Start Small

Always see the solution (or the end result or the outcome) as a matter of causes and effects that interact dynamically over time (that is, a web of causation).[1] To begin, contemplate the web in its entirety, but start by measuring only a few key, high-leverage causal elements (process and case mix variables) and one or two critical outcomes. As time passes, data on more of the system variables (inputs, processes, outputs, feedback loops) can be captured for learning, reflection, and taking action.

2. More Data Are Not Necessarily Better Data: Seek Usefulness, Not Perfection, in Measures

Be clear about what question must be answered and then target data collection to find the answer. More data are not necessarily better data. Collecting more data than needed incurs many risks: The work of collection might preclude cooperation from those who have to do it, more data might yield more collection and recording errors, data collection can be expensive, and finally, the importance of the effort might be compromised if those for whom it is to provide help regard these measures as irrelevant. Discontinue measures when it is determined that new measures are more useful.

3. Write Down the Operational Definitions of Measures

The quality of measurement values is contingent on the accuracy of the individual data elements. Having and following clear operational definitions is essential for recording data and creating measures if the data are to be reliable and valid. In addition, interpreting data is easier when documented definitions are readily available. When using a newly created data collection form, make full use of self-coding data sheets that reflect the operational definition in the layout of the question and in the response choices and that also have operational definitions printed on the front or back side of the data collection form.

4. Use a Balanced Set of Input, Process, Outcome, and Cost Measures

To gain insight, it is necessary to deepen one's understanding of the web of causation. This involves capturing sources of causation (inputs), intervening events (processes), and transitions in important results (outcomes and costs) of the system that is to be managed and improved. Instrument panels provide critical, real-time information on the system's total performance and can prompt the user to make wise decisions and, if necessary, make rapid midcourse corrections.[2] The use of inclusive frameworks (such as structure-process-outcome, value compass thinking, and microsystem approaches) can help reveal which parts of the system are important for measurement and which interactions between parts are most variable and critical.

5. Build Measurement into Daily Work and Job Descriptions

Data collection, analysis, and display should be designed into the flow of medical practice. Measurement is already built into some clinical practice routines—for example, taking vital signs at the beginning of an office visit or cardiac monitoring of patients in coronary care units. New measurements can be designed into clinical care routines and into the job descriptions of people who are involved in the care of patients. The key idea is to capture the right data, correctly, and to use them immediately and repeatedly.

6. Use Quantitative and Qualitative Data

Quantitative data can provide limited and precise views of how the system is performing and how the patient is doing. Maps of causes and effects and of feedback loops can also provide a sense of how different measures interrelate. Quantitative data provide a simplified model of reality. Qualitative data (observations, critical incidents, verbatim comments, unsolicited compliments and complaints) can provide a richer understanding of the underlying background from which the quantitative data emerge.

7. Use Available Data, if Possible; Otherwise, Measure Small Representative Samples

All systems are constantly producing data that can be used for learning, managing, researching, and taking action. Sometimes the data produced by the system are already being captured with sufficient accuracy (both valid and reliable), and what needs to be done is to retrieve, analyze, and display the data in a useful manner. If the data exist and are sufficiently accurate, use them. Many times, however, the question that is posed cannot be answered by reprocessing captured data. Under these conditions, new data must be gathered prospectively. In this case, begin by gathering data on small, representative, time-ordered samples. Using a systematic or random sample—or selecting a judgment sample—to reflect how the system is performing under different known conditions can be helpful.

8. Display Key Measures (for Viewing by Staff and Patients) That Demonstrate Trends over Time

Data are not self-actuating; they must be analyzed, displayed, and interpreted to create the conditions for taking intelligent action. Graphic visual displays of data can help people interpret results and create the conditions for taking such action. Consider building viewable "data walls" or "storyboards" to create a physical, visual environment through which data can be communicated in a timely manner. One of the most powerful ways for displaying data is to use statistical process control methods. Graphically tracking results—or drivers of results—can help us gain insight to inform appropriate action on the basis of historical trends, current values, and thus probable future outcomes.

9. Develop a Measurement Team and Establish Ownership

Sharing the burden of measurement lightens the load for everyone. Understanding and participation can be broadened by inviting key people, with different professional skills and training, to take responsibility for various facets of data collection and analysis. In general, a small group of interested people is needed to create a data environment that will be most useful to members of the microsystem who work together to deliver medical care. This small measurement team can develop operational definitions and data management plans, which can be reviewed by the entire staff and by patients for consensus and implementation.

For a more detailed review of these principles, please see Nelson EC, et al. Using data to improve medical practice by measuring processes and outcomes of care. *Jt Comm J Qual Improv.* 2000 Dec;26(12):667–685.

Guidelines for Designing a Measurement Process: A 12-Pack of Suggestions

Aim, Users, Uses

1. Ensure that the intended use and analysis of data are clear.

2. Ensure that the methods of organizing, displaying, and summarizing data allow study of factors that might have important effects on the results.

Definitions

3. Develop clear definitions of how observations are to be translated into measurements or evaluations.

4. Ensure that the method of measurement results in obtaining the intended information.

5. Ensure that the measurement methods to be used are clear and simple and minimize on-the-spot decision making.

Planning

6. Design measurement that isn't too big—remember, "less is more."

7. Embed measurement and data collection into the daily activities of the system under study.

8. Ensure that measurement and data analysis are timely.

9. Develop a plan for training those who will make the measurements, record the data, and keep a diary for recording auxiliary information.

10. Perform pilot studies of definitions, methods of measurement, data collection forms, and training.

11. Determine who is responsible for the measurement process.

12. Inform all affected associates about the purpose of collecting data.

References

1. MacMahon B, Pugh TF. *Epidemiology: Principles and Methods.* Boston: Little, Brown, 1970.
2. Nelson EC, et al. Report cards or instrument panels: Who needs what? *Jt Comm J Qual Improv.* 1995 Apr;21(4):155–166.

Appendix E

Web-Based Quality and Safety Resources

Mary A. Dolansky

The Internet is a dynamic and evolving resource for information, ideas, and useful tools that can facilitate practice-based learning and improvement. Specific websites might be helpful to individuals who wish to do the following:

- Improve health care
- Develop practice-based learning groups
- Scan the literature for benchmarking data and evidence-based best practices
- Identify clinical practice guidelines and quality metrics
- Create survey instruments to assess local performance
- Dig more deeply into sources of information and knowledge

In Table E-1, below, we provide a small starter set of websites that are useful for one or more of these purposes. This list is certainly not exhaustive but is representative of websites that the editors have found useful for initiation of improvement projects. The sites are listed alphabetically.

Table E-1. Starter Set of Quality and Safety Websites

Organization or Resource	Web Address	Description
Accreditation Council for Graduate Medical Education (ACGME)	http://www.acgme.org/acgmeweb	An accreditation agency that advances the quality of resident physicians' education through accreditation
Agency for Healthcare Research and Quality (AHRQ) AHRQ Patient Safety Tools and Resources	http://www.ahrq.gov/qual/pstools.pdf	A collection of free resources and tools for health care organizations, providers, and policy makers to improve patient safety in health care settings
AHRQ WebM&M: Morbidity and Mortality Rounds on the Web	http://www.webmm.ahrq.gov	A database of cases in which an error was committed, including commentary on how to prevent the situation in the future
Baldrige Performance Excellence Program	http://www.nist.gov/baldrige	A program that attempts to improve the competiveness and performance of organizations by encouraging performance excellence
The Dartmouth Institute Microsystem Academy Clinical Microsystems	http://www.clinicalmicrosystem.org	An academy that provides resources and training to help improve the care of patients

continued on next page

Table E-1. Starter Set of Quality and Safety Websites, *continued*

Organization or Resource	Web Address	Description
5 Million Lives campaign of the Institute for Healthcare Improvement	http://www.ihi.org/offerings/Initiatives/ PastStrategicInitiatives/5MillionLives Campaign/Pages/default.aspx	A campaign that supported and provided guidelines for the improvement of medical care in the United States
Hospital Compare, US Department of Health and Human Services	http://www.hospitalcompare.hhs.gov	A resource that allows patients to compare hospitals and find the best institution at which to receive care
HowsYourHealth	http://www.howsyourhealth.org	A website that helps older patients make decisions about their health care
Ideal Micropractice	http://www.idealmicropractice.com	A blog that discusses health treatments and ways to stay healthier
Institute for Safe Medication Practices	http://www.ismp.org	An organization that is devoted to medication error prevention and safe medication use
Institute of Medicine (IOM)	http://www.iom.edu	An independent organization that provides unbiased advice to decision makers and the public
Intermountain Healthcare (IHC)	http://intermountainhealthcare.org/ qualityandresearch/institute/courses/ atp/Pages/home.aspx	An Advanced Training Program (ATP) that covers quality improvement, outcome measurement, and management of both clinical and nonclinical processes
Joint Commission Resources	http://www.jcrinc.com	A collection of resources—including publications, education resources, consultation, and evaluation services—aimed at improving safety and quality of health care
Medical Office Survey on Patient Safety Culture	http://www.ahrq.gov/qual/mosurvey08/ medoffsurv.htm	A survey given to health care providers that can be used to improve patient safety and quality of care
National Patient Safety Goals	www.jointcommission.org/patientsafety/ nationalpatientsafetygoals	Set of Joint Commission requirements to promote specific improvements in patient safety that highlight problematic areas in health care and describe evidence-based and expert-based solutions to these problems
National Quality Measures Clearinghouse	http://www.qualitymeasures.ahrq.gov	An agency that provides measures currently being used by the division in the US Department of Health and Human Services for quality measurement, improvement, and reporting
Patient Safety and Quality	http://www.ahrq.gov/qual/nurseshdbk	An evidence-based handbook for nurses to enhance patient outcomes
Patient Safety Glossary	http://webmm.ahrq.gov/popup_ glossary.aspx	A glossary that defines terminology in medical error and patient safety literature

continued on next page

Table E-1. Starter Set of Quality and Safety Websites, *continued*

Organization or Resource	Web Address	Description
Safety Climate Survey	http://www.uth.tmc.edu/schools/med/imed/patient_safety/documents/Survey-Safety-Climate-EWR.pdf	An survey to assess the safety climate in clinical practice
Sentinel Event Datbase	http:www.jointcommission.org/sentinel_event.aspx	An aggregated collection of sentinel event-related data, reported to The Joint Commission from its accredited organizations, that help The Joint Commission identify causes, trends, settings, and outcomes of sentinel events for which it can provide critical information in the prevention of such sentinel events to accredited health care organizations and the public
Serious Reportable Events	http://www.qualityforum.org/Topics/SREs/Serious_Reportable_Events.aspx	A list of extremely rare events that should never happen to a patient
Society for General Internal Medicine	http://www.sgim.org/aclgim-tools-programs/quality-portfolio	A portfolio that provides a framework and samples for quality improvement
University of California, San Francisco QI Portfolio for Academic Advancement	http://medicine.ucsf.edu/safety/overview/portfolio.html	A resource designed to better capture the activities and accomplishments of faculty engaged in quality improvement work, regardless of whether it is their career focus
US Department of Veterans Affairs National Center for Patient Safety (VA NCPS)	http://www.patientsafety.gov	A center to support the nationwide reduction and prevention of inadvertent harm to patients as a result of their care
US National Library of Medicine (NLM)	http://www.nlm.nih.gov	A collection of resources that covers a broad range of medical topics in a variety of formats

Appendix F

SUPPLEMENTS TO CHAPTER 8

Programs Used by Kaiser Permanente to Enhance Quality and Team-Based Care

Connie Lopez, Michael A. Tijerina

The following supplementary information goes along with each of the programs listed in Chapter 8, Table 8-4 (page 105).

Collaborating for Outcomes:
• Figure F-1. RN–MD Report-Out Tool

National Critical Events Team Training—Simulation Instructor (Level I) Course:
• Figure F-2. Sample Course Agenda for Critical Events Team Training (CETT): Train-the-Trainer
• Figure F-3. Course Surveys
• Figure F-4. Crisis Resource Management (CRM) Observation Tool

National Simulation-Based Education and Training— Simulation Instructor (Level II) Course:
• Figure F-5. Sample Course Agenda for National Simulation Based Education and Training Level II: Train-the-Trainer

National Perinatal Patient Safety Programs:
• Figure F-6. Sample Course Objectives and Agenda and Objectives for National Perinatal Safety Programs
• Figure F-7. Knowledge and Skills Checklist: Vacuum Delivery—Provider
• Figure F-8. Knowledge and Skills Checklist: Vacuum Delivery—RN
• Figure F-9. Knowledge and Skills Checklist: Shoulder Dystocia Delivery—Provider
• Figure F-10. Knowledge and Skills Checklist: Shoulder Dystocia Delivery—RN

Table F-1. Teamwork and Quality Improvement Resources

Table F-2. Tools to Assess Teamwork and Collaboration

Figure F-1. RN–MD Report-Out Tool

1a. Department (Team)			
1b. Key Contact	Name: Email: Phone:	1c. Team Members:	
2. Existing Initiative (i.e., Projects / Programs)		**3. Organizational Alignment**	
		❑ Quality & Safety ❑ Service ❑ Resource Stewardship	❑ People: Best Place to Work ❑ Patient Care Experience ❑ Other: _____
4. Flashpoint & Flashpoint Drivers		**5. Small First Steps**	
Identify Flashpoint (challenge/barrier): Describe Flashpoint Drivers: (Communication, Competency, Process, Roles, Resources)			
6. Potential Outcomes		**7. Plan for Information Sharing**	
		Identify forums for sharing information with other RNs and MDs (e.g., staff meetings, huddles, UBTs, physician lounges, break rooms)	

RN–MD Report-Out Tool Exercise Instructions

STEP 1 Sit with colleagues from your team (department, workgroup, unit-based-team [UBT])	• Write down the (1a) department (team name), (1b) key contact, (1c) team members.

STEP 2: Existing Initiatives (Projects, Programs)	• Review the list of existing initiatives for your team or medical center area.
	• Pick one initiative your group will use as the focus for this exercise.
	    — Suggested criteria:
	        • Current initiative the team is working on right now.
	        • Data or information about the initiative is available.
	• The team has encountered some challenges due to relationship or collaboration challenges.

STEP 3: Organizational Alignment	• Identify the organizational alignment . . . what area(s) is the initiative impacting?
STEP 4: Flashpoint & Flashpoint Drivers	• Describe one flashpoint (challenge/barrier) currently being experienced within this initiative. • Describe the possible underlying drivers for the flashpoint.
STEP 5: Small First Steps	• Discuss and agree on actions this group can take within the next 30 days.
STEP 6: Potential Outcomes	• Describe what the initiative will look like if the flashpoint driver is addressed and resolved.
STEP 7: Plan for Information Sharing	• Identify how you will share your learning from today and the Report-Out Tool with the rest of your team members and colleagues in your department.

Figure F-2. Sample Course Agenda for Critical Events Team Training (CETT): Train-the-Trainer

AGENDA – DAY 1		
Time	**Topic**	**Presenter**
7:30 am – 8:00 am	Breakfast Welcome and Introductions • Expectations & Goals	National Instructors
8:00 am – 9:00 am	Why We Rehearse/Setting the Stage • Learner-centric Education	National Instructors
9:00 am – 9:15 am	Break	
9:15 am – 10:00 am	"Turning a Team of Experts into an Expert Team"	
10:00 am – 11:45 am	Pre-Simulation Survey Meet the "Patients" (Sim Family) Simulation Debrief Simulation Post-Simulation Survey	National Instructors
11:45 am – 12:15 pm	Lunch	
12:15 pm – 1:15 pm	Teaching Methods & Activities (PART I) • Types/Moulage	National Instructors
1:15 pm – 1:45 pm	Teaching Methods & Activities (PART II) • Objectives • Scenario Writing	National Instructors
1:45 pm – 2:00 pm	Break	
2:00 pm – 3:00 pm	Training to Outcomes • Scenario Writing Activity • Metrics/Tool Development	National Instructors
3:00 pm – 4:45 pm	Debriefing • Three-step Process • Table Top Exercise • Video Exercise	National Instructors
4:45 pm – 5:00 pm	Wrap-up	National Instructors

continued on next page

Figure F-2. Sample Course Agenda for Critical Events Team Training (CETT): Train-the-Trainer, *continued*

AGENDA – DAY 2		
Time	**Topic**	**Presenter**
7:30 am – 8:00 am	Breakfast Review of Day 1	
8:00 am – 9:00 am	Equipment & Moulage Stations	Equipment Specialists National Instructors
9:00 am – 10:00 am	Set up and Practice for Simulations	Teams
10:00 am – 10:15 am	Break	
10:15 am – 10:30 am	Meet the Patients	New Trainers: Team 1
10:30 am – 11:00 am	Simulation 1	New Trainers: Team 1
11:00 am – 11:30 am	Debrief Simulation 1	New Trainers: Team 1
11:30 am – 12:15 pm	Lunch	
12:15 pm – 12:30 pm	Set up Simulation 2	New Trainers: Team 2
12:30 pm – 12:45 pm	Meet the Patients	New Trainers: Team 2
12:45 pm – 1:15 pm	Simulation 2	New Trainers: Team 2
1:15 pm – 1:45 pm	Debrief Simulation 2	New Trainers: Team 2
1:45 pm – 2:00 pm	Break	
2:00 pm – 3:00 pm	The Practical Side of Running CETT	Teams
3:00 pm – 4:45 pm	Set up for Simulations on Day 3	Teams
4:45 pm – 5:00 pm	Debrief the Day	Teams

continued on next page

Figure F-2. Sample Course Agenda for Critical Events Team Training (CETT): Train-the-Trainer, *continued*

AGENDA – DAY 3 *(PM sessions structured in same way for Team 2)*		
Time	**Topic**	**Presenter**
7:30 am – 8:00 am	Breakfast	
8:00 am – 8:10 am	Welcome and Introductions	New Trainers Team 1
8:10 am – 8:20 am	Pre-Simulation Survey	New Trainers Team 1
8:20 am – 8:30 am	Review Objectives for the Day Overview of Attendee Binder	New Trainers Team 1
8:30 am – 9:15 am	"Turning a Team of Experts into an Expert Team"	New Trainers Team 1
9:15 am – 9:30 am	Meet the Patients	New Trainers Team 1
9:30 am – 10:00 am	Simulation 1	New Trainers Team 1
10:00 am – 10:30 am	Debrief for Simulation 1	New Trainers Team 1
10:30 am – 10:45 am	Break	
10:45 am – 11:15 am	Simulation 2	New Trainers Team 1
11:15 am – 11:45 am	Debrief for Simulation 2	New Trainers Team 1
11:45 am – 11:50 am	Closing Comments	New Trainers Team 1
11:50 am – 12:00 noon	Post-Simulation Survey	New Trainers Team 1

Figure F-3. Course Surveys

Pre- and Post-Course Survey for Critical Events Team Training (CETT)

CRITICAL EVENTS TEAM TRAINING
Pre-Simulation Survey Questions

Circle the number from the Response Scale that best rates your opinion for this Critical Event Team Training.	Response Scale			
	4	3	2	1
	Agree		Disagree	
I am prepared to technically respond proficiently during critical events.	4	3	2	1
I understand my role as part of the team in this critical event.	4	3	2	1
Our team communication is good leading to stronger team performance for this critical event.	4	3	2	1
I feel comfortable communicating with my team members during this critical event.	4	3	2	1
My unit is a "high-reliability"* unit. *an environment where safety is the highest priority, where there is preoccupation with what could fail, open environment to discuss error, everyone encouraged to speak up about hazards, rewards for safe actions, <u>training for hazardous situations</u>	4	3	2	1

Post-Simulation Survey Questions

Circle the number from the Response Scale that best rates your opinion for this Critical Event Team Training.	Response Scale			
	4	3	2	1
	Agree		Disagree	
I am **MORE** prepared to technically respond proficiently to this critical event.	4	3	2	1
I understand my role as part of the team in this critical event	4	3	2	1
Our team communication is good leading to stronger team performance for this critical event.	4	3	2	1
I feel **MORE** comfortable communicating with my team members during this critical event.	4	3	2	1
My unit is a "high-reliability"* unit. *an environment where safety is the highest priority, where there is preoccupation with what could fail, open environment to discuss error, everyone encouraged to speak up about hazards, rewards for safe actions, <u>training for hazardous situations</u>	4	3	2	1

Figure F-4. Crisis Resource Management (CRM) Observation Tool

Code Observation Sheet Used for Simulation Training and Clinical Events

COMMUNICATION	Yes	No	Inconsistent	NA
Is Leader evident?				
Title: If not MD, is an MD present?				
Do people announce themselves?				
Does Leader assign roles?				
Does Leader give directed directions?				
Is there transparent thinking?				
Is there closed loop communication?				
Is there SBAR to orient new members?				
Role clarity?				
SITUATIONAL AWARENESS	**Yes**	**No**	**Inconsistent**	**NA**
Is there resource allocation?				
Is there task fixation?				
Does Leader ensure high-quality CPR is in progress?				
Does Leader assure the airway is being managed appropriately?				
Are there people in the room not doing anything?				
Does Leader use a "global" vs. "local" perspective?				
DECISION MAKING	**Yes**	**No**	**Inconsistent**	**NA**
Anticipate and plan?				
Distribution of workload?				
OTHER	**Yes**	**No**	**Inconsistent**	**NA**
Knowledge of equipment?				
Patient centered care?				
Documentation (during code)?				
Hand-off using SBAR at end of code (if survives)?				
Hand-off using SBAR at end of code (if patient doesn't survive)?				
Medication Verbal Order Read Back?				
Debrief after code?				
Number of people?				
COMMENTS:				

Data collected includes date; time code called & ended; location, and time of observer arrival

Based on Crisis Resource Management (CRM). CPR: cardio pulmonary resuscitation. SBAR: Situation, Background, Assessment, Recommendation.

Figure F-5. Sample Course Agenda for National Simulation Based Education and Training Level II: Train-the-Trainer

AGENDA – DAY 1		
Time	**Topic**	**Presenter**
7:30 am – 8:00 am	Breakfast	
8:00 am – 8:15 am	Welcome and Introductions	National Instructors
8:15 am – 9:15 am	Setting the Stage • Expectations & Goals • Foundations of Practice • Learner-Centric Education	National Instructors
9:15 am – 10:00 am	Program Overview • Program Design & Planning	National Instructors
10:00 am – 10:15 am	Break	
10:15 am – 11:45 am	Teaching Methods & Activities (PART I) • Types & Tools	National Instructors
11:45 am – 12:30 pm	Lunch	
12:30 pm – 2:30 pm	Teaching Methods & Activities (PART II) • Instructional Design • Objectives • Scenario Writing	National Instructors
2:30 pm – 2:45 pm	Break	
2:45 pm – 4:30 pm	Training to Outcomes • Metrics • Tool Development	National Instructors
4:30 pm – 5:00 pm	Debriefing/Jeopardy	Teams

continued on next page

Figure F-5. Sample Course Agenda for National Simulation Based Education and Training Level II: Train-the-Trainer, *continued*

AGENDA – DAY 2		
Time	**Topic**	**Presenter**
7:30 am – 8:00 am	Breakfast	
8:00 am – 10:00 am	Enhancing Performance and Patient Safety: (TeamSTEPPS)	National Instructors
10:00 am – 10:15 am	Break	
10:15 am – 11:30 am	Enhancing Performance and Patient Safety (TeamSTEPPS)	National Instructors
11:30 am – 12:15 pm	Lunch	
12:15 pm – 1:15 pm	Group 1 – Setting the Stage: Special Effects	Group 2 – Technology: Video & Data Collection
1:15 pm – 2:15 pm	Group 1 - Technology: Video & Data Collection	Group 2 – Setting the Stage: Special Effects
2:15 pm – 2:30 pm	Break	
2:30 pm – 3:30 pm	Technology: Advanced Programming for Simulation Equipment	Teams
3:30 pm – 4:30 pm	Set-up for Simulations on Day 3	Teams
4:30 pm – 5:00 pm	Debriefing	Teams

continued on next page

TeamSTEPPS: Team Strategies & Tools to Enhance Performance & Patient Safety.

Figure F-5. Sample Course Agenda for National Simulation Based Education and Training Level II: Train-the-Trainer, *continued*

AGENDA – DAY 3		
Time	**Topic**	**Presenter**
7:30 am – 8:00 am	Breakfast	
8:00 am – 10:30 am	Debriefing & Guidelines for Improving Effectiveness • Three-step process	National Instructor
10:30 am – 10:45 am	Break	
10:45 am – 12:15 am	Group Practice • Table Top Exercise • Video Exercise	Teams
12:15 pm – 1:00 pm	Lunch	
1:00 pm – 1:15 pm	Introduction & Simulation 1	Teams
1:15 pm – 1:45 pm	Debrief & Summary for Sim 1	Teams
1:45 pm – 2:15 pm	Debrief New Debriefers	Teams
2:15 pm – 2:30 pm	Break	
2:30 pm – 2:45 pm	Introduction & Simulation 2	Teams
2:45 pm – 3:15 pm	Debrief & Summary for Sim 2	Teams
3:15 pm – 3:45 pm	Debrief New Debriefers	Teams
3:45 pm – 4:00 pm	Break	
4:00 pm – 4:15 pm	Evaluation & Survey	National Instructors
4:15pm – 5:00 pm	Feedback and Next Steps	Teams

Figure F-6. Sample Course Objectives and Agenda for National Perinatal Safety Programs

Objectives for Vacuum Delivery
1. Identify obstetrical factors that influence the outcome of a vacuum delivery
2. Cite indications and contraindications for a vacuum delivery
3. Describe anatomical principles, clinical reasoning, and technical skills required for the safe use of a vacuum
4. Compare and contrast the efficacy of the vacuum products available
5. Identify when to abandon the vacuum procedure
Objectives for Shoulder Dystocia Delivery
6. Identify risk factors for shoulder dystocia
7. Identify complications of shoulder dystocia
8. Describe maneuvers for emergent management of shoulder dystocia
9. Demonstrate medical simulation of shoulder dystocia
Objectives for Perinatal fetal heart rate (FHR) Assessment and Response
1. Understand the importance of Standardized Language (NICHD; National Institute of Child Health and Human Development)
2. Describe the significance of baseline variability
3. Discern Emergent and Urgent FHR patterns

TIME	TOPIC	FACILITATOR
8:00	Welcome	RN/MD
8:05	Why are we here? • Med legal/risk data	National Risk Director
8:35	Why Standardized and skill & Team-based Training?	Regional Risk Management
8:45	Human Factors Review • Communication • Common Language for Briefing 　— Shoulder dystocia 　— Vacuum • Teamwork and roles • Standardized alert system	RN/MD
9:10	Didactic: Shoulder dystocia & Vacuum delivery • Perinatal FHR Assessment and Response	MD/CNM Regional Risk Management
10:20	**BREAK**	
10:30	Expert Team Modeling: Shoulder dystocia & Vacuum delivery	Physician
10:45	Introduction to the equipment & Hands-on **[names of proprietary equipment removed]**	Participants
11:05	CETT Scenario #1 and Debriefing	Participants
11:30	CETT Scenario #2 and Debriefing	Participants
11:55 – 12:15	Wrap-up, Post test & Evaluations	RN/MD

Figure F-7. Knowledge and Skills Checklist: Vacuum Delivery—Provider

PERFORMANCE CRITERIA – The following measures are to be taken by a <u>Provider</u> upon decision to perform a vacuum delivery	MET	NOT MET
1. Makes diagnosis and clearly states intent to perform vacuum delivery		
2. Informs patient and family of risks, benefits, and alternative options		
3. Asks RN to request nursing assistance and to notify neonatal team		
4. States plan: criteria for when to stop vacuum attempts		
5. Applies vacuum at flexion point, using constant smooth traction in the axis of pelvis, without rotational or side to side movements, during maternal pushing effort		
6. Abandons procedure if > 2 pop-offs, lack of descent with each pull, or if delivery not imminent after 3 pulls or > 20 minutes (pull = contractions)		
7. If traction measured, uses < 25 lbs		
8. Does not attempt forceps pull if vacuum fails (forceps pull ≠ pull)		
9. Describes appropriate documentation		

Figure F-8. Knowledge and Skills Checklist: Vacuum Delivery—RN

PERFORMANCE CRITERIA – The following measures are to be taken by the <u>Primary RN</u> (maternal responsibility) for vacuum delivery	MET	NOT MET
1. If using a *Mityvac*, assists with maintaining suction		
2. Records time when vacuum pressure applied		
3. Records number of disengagements or "pop-offs"		
4. Informs physician if > 2 pop-offs occurs		
5. Informs physician when 10 of accrued time at max pressure		
6. Alert to lack of descent with 3 consecutive tractions (pulls)		
7. Uses: Stop-the-Line code word if > 2 pop-offs, lack of descent with each pull, or if delivery not imminent after 3 tractions (pulls) or > 20 minutes		
8. Assists in maintaining external FHR monitor as needed		
9. Preps patient for c/sec		
PERFORMANCE CRITERIA – The following measures are to be taken by the <u>Second RN</u> (neonatal responsibility) for a vacuum delivery	MET	NOT MET
1. Maintains surveillance of fetal heart tracing		
2. Ensures documentation of vacuum delivery is occurring		
3. Prepares for the potential of a shoulder dystocia		
4. Provides SBAR briefing to team that arrives to provide assistance		
5. Receives infant after delivery if NICU team not present		
6. Notifies NICU team as needed		
7. Stays with primary nurse until excused		
PERFORMANCE CRITERIA – The following measures are to be taken by the <u>Charge RN</u> upon failure of vacuum delivery		
1. Ensures that all staff are notified if transfer to OR for C/sec		
2. Assists with family as needed		
3. Assists with transfer to the OR		

SBAR: Situation, Background, Assessment, Recommendation. NICU: neonatal intensive care unit.

Figure F-9. Knowledge and Skills Checklist: Shoulder Dystocia Delivery—Provider

PERFORMANCE CRITERIA – The following measures are to be taken by the <u>Provider</u> for shoulder dystocia delivery	MET	NOT MET
Appropriate Delegation / Communication		
1. Call the Emergency – Request Physician Assistance		
2. Explain to patient briefly what the problem is and importance of following directions closely		
3. Remind patient not to push until requested to do so		
4. Update physician help when entering the room, and what maneuvers attempted so far		
5. Call out the delivery of head		
6. Call each maneuver as attempted		
Appropriate Management of Clinical Maneuvers		
7. Patient buttocks moved to edge (end) of bed		
8. **Call for McRoberts Maneuver**: Apply traction while patient pushes		
9. If McRoberts alone is not successful, **Call for Suprapubic Pressure**: Continue downward traction while patient pushes		
10. If unsuccessful, **consider episiotomy** if it will make internal maneuvers easier. Communicate with patient decision.		
11. Call out that you are attempting **Delivery of Posterior Arm**		
12. If unsuccessful, Call out that you are **Performing Internal Rotation Maneuvers and to STOP Suprapubic Pressure**		
13. If unsuccessful, Call out that you want a **Gaskins Maneuver**: Assist rolling patient over into an all fours position. Not appropriate if patient has a dense epidural.		
14. If unsuccessful consider **Cleidotomy**		
15. If unsuccessful consider **Zavanelli Maneuver and call a Code C**		
Debrief		
What went well?		
What could have been improved?		
What needs to be worked on?		

Note: Kaiser Permanente does not endorse the use of any particular products.

Figure F-10. Knowledge and Skills Checklist: Shoulder Dystocia Delivery—RN

PERFORMANCE CRITERIA – The following measures are to be taken by the <u>Primary RN</u> upon discovery of a shoulder dystocia prior to delivery	MET	NOT MET
1. Marks time when requested by provider		
2. Requests help as needed or instructed		
3. Gets stepstool and positions the patient and bed		
4. Assists with McRoberts and suprapubic pressure on request		
5. Stops suprapubic pressure with rotational maneuvers or delivery of posterior arm as instructed by provider		
6. Calls out each minute interval from "mark time" to delivery of baby		
7. Maintains external heart rate monitoring		
8. Does not use fundal pressure		
PERFORMANCE CRITERIA – The following measures are to be taken by the <u>Second RN</u> upon discovery of a shoulder dystocia prior to delivery	MET	NOT MET
1. Ensures stepstool is in place (if not already done by primary RN)		
2. Provides assistance with McRoberts and suprapubic pressure as directed by provider		
3. Assists in maintaining external FHR monitor as needed		
4. Provides SBAR briefing to team that arrives to provide assistance		
5. Receives infant after delivery if NICU team not present		
6. Assists NICU team as needed		
7. Stays with primary nurse until excused		
PERFORMANCE CRITERIA – The following measures are to be taken by the <u>Charge RN</u> upon discovery of a shoulder dystocia prior to delivery		
1. Ensures that all staff required are present		
2. Assists as necessary with delivery or as directed by provider		
3. Assists with family as needed		
4. Clears space for OB and NICU staff in delivery room		

SBAR: Situation, Background, Assessment, Recommendation. FHR: fetal heart rate. NICU: neonatal intensive care unit.

Teamwork and Quality Improvement Resources for Frontline Staff and Staff/Faculty Development

Maryjoan D. Ladden, Carlos A. Estrada

Table F-1. Teamwork and Quality Improvement Resources

Program Name and Description	Contact Information	Benefits
For Frontline Staff		
TeamSTEPPS A program and tools to enhance team performance and improve patient safety that has three phases: assessment; planning and implementation; and sustainment.	Developed by the US Department of Defense and the Agency for Healthcare Research and Quality (AHRQ). http://teamstepps.ahrq.gov/	Standardized curriculum that can be adapted for target audience and environment. No cost for materials. Requires buy-in from leadership.
Transforming Care at the Bedside (TCAB) A package of resources designed to empower and prepare frontline staff to improve care delivery at the bedside. Resources include a primer/toolkit to redesign work processes; and a guide to improve strategic communication across clinical and support staff.	Developed by the Institute for Healthcare Improvement (IHI) through a grant from the Robert Wood Johnson Foundation (RWJF). http://www.ihi.org/offerings/Initiatives/PastStrategicInitiatives/TCAB/Pages/default.aspx	Tested in many hospitals across the United States. No cost for materials. Can be used by both frontline staff and managers. Requires buy-in from leadership.
How to Use SBAR, Advocacy and Team Behaviors to Improve Patient Outcomes A seven-page scenario, with debriefing opportunities, designed to identify opportunities to improve communication in care of postoperative patient.	Developed for teaching purposes by The University of California, San Francisco (UCSF) School of Medicine. http://medschool.ucsf.edu/gme/pdf/MDRNcommunicationfacilitatorguide.pdf	Very relatable scenario that can be used both for frontline staff and for teaching purposes. No cost for materials.
Culture Clues™ **University of Washington Medical Center** Culture Clues™ are tip sheets for clinicians, designed to increase awareness about concepts and preferences of patients from diverse cultures.	Developed by Patient and Family Education Services at the University of Washington Medical Center. http://depts.washington.edu/pfes/CultureClues.htm	Available for a variety of cultures. No cost for materials. Can be immediately used with patients.
For Staff/Faculty Development		
Quality and Safety Education for Nurses (QSEN) Many resources, including videos and curricula, to teach the knowledge, skills, and attitudes for each of the QSEN competencies: patient-centered care, teamwork and collaboration, evidence-based practice, quality improvement, safety, informatics.	Developed by the QSEN team at University of North Carolina at Chapel Hill and national consultants through a grant from the Robert Wood Johnson Foundation. http://www.qsen.org	Helps bridge the gap between academic education and nursing practice. Designed for nursing education but can be easily adapted for interprofessional use. No cost for materials.

continued on next page

Table F-1. Teamwork and Quality Improvement Resources, *continued*

Program Name and Description	Contact Information	Benefits
Patient Safety Tools: Improving Safety at the Point of Care (AHRQ) Seventeen toolkits that contain a variety of evidence-based tools, including training materials, medication guides, and checklists that can be adapted to other institutions and care settings.	Developed under AHRQ's Partnerships in Implementing Patient Safety (PIPS) grant program. http://www.ahrq.gov/qual/pips	Developed in the field and designed to be implemented by multidisciplinary users. No cost for materials.
Patient Safety Glossary (AHRQ) A glossary of quality and safety terms with definitions that enjoy the widest use.	Developed by the Agency for Healthcare Research and Quality (AHRQ). http://webmm.ahrq.gov/popup_glossary.aspx	Standardized definitions of common quality improvement and safety terms. Can be used to facilitate team and organizational communication. No cost for materials.
Advances in Patient Safety: From Research to Implementation A collection of articles and useful tools and products that can be used to improve patient safety.	Developed by the Agency for Healthcare Research and Quality (AHRQ) and the Department of Defense - Health Affairs. http://www.ahrq.gov/qual/advances	References and tools applicable to a variety of clinical settings and patient populations. No cost for materials.
Achieving Competence Today (ACT) A self-directed modular action learning curriculum on CD designed to teach about systems and practice improvement.	Developed by Partnerships for Quality Education through a grant from the Robert Wood Johnson Foundation. http://www.rwjf.org	Can be used for interprofessional learners and staff to work together around quality and safety. Tested in many academic health centers across the United States. No cost for materials.
World Health Organization (WHO) Patient Safety Curriculum Guide A 270-page guide that includes a curriculum for teachers and also checklists for clinicians to monitor safety issues in the hospital setting.	Developed by the World Health Organization. http://www.who.int/patientsafety/education/curriculum/en/index.html	Ready-to-teach, topic-based patient safety programs for 11 safety topics that can be used as a whole or for any of the topics alone. No cost for materials.
Medical Teamwork and Patient Safety: The Evidence-Based Relation A report presenting the evidence on relevant team training programs from aviation and other domains as well as an evaluation of current health care team training initiatives.	Developed by American Institutes for Research, University of Central Florida, and the University of Miami Center for Patient Safety through a grant from AHRQ. http://www.ahrq.gov/qual/medteam	Useful review of what we know about the effectiveness of team training programs. No cost for materials.
US Veterans Affairs (VA) National Quality Scholars Fellowship Program A two-year interprofessional fellowship program to apply health care improvement methods to the care of veterans, teach health professionals about health care improvement, and perform research and develop new knowledge for the ongoing improvement of the quality and value of health care services.	The Veterans Health Administration created VAQS, the VA National Quality Scholars Fellowship Program, in Collaboration with The Dartmouth Institute for Health Policy and Clinical Practice (TDI). http://www.vaqs.org	Open to board-certified physicians and nurses pursuing or having completed doctoral education. At nine sites across the United States and Canada.

Tools to Assess Teamwork and Collaboration

Carlos A. Estrada, Maryjoan D. Ladden

Table F-2. Tools to Assess Teamwork and Collaboration

Assessment Tool	Description	How to Access and Use It
TeamSTEPPS™ Teamwork Attitudes Questionnaire (T-TAQ)	Determines whether TeamSTEPPS tools and strategies enhanced an individual participant's attitudes toward teamwork, increased knowledge about effective team practice, and improved team skills. Tool can be used to assess specific needs within the unit or health care institution and whether the intervention produced the desired attitude change. Measures individual *attitudes* related to team functioning: team structure, leadership, situation monitoring, mutual support, and communication (30 items).	T-TAQ Manual. http://teamstepps.ahrq.gov/taq_index.htm Agency for Healthcare Research and Quality. TeamSTEPPS®: National Implementation. 2010. Accessed Oct 20, 2012. http://teamstepps.ahrq.gov. Clancy CM, Tornberg DN. TeamSTEPPS: Assuring optimal teamwork in clinical settings. *Am J Med Qual.* 2007 May–Jun;22(3):214–217.
TeamSTEPPS™ Teamwork Perceptions Questionnaire (T-TPQ)	Determines how an individual perceives the current state of teamwork within an organization. T-TPQ correlates with patient safety domains. Measures individual *perceptions* related to team functioning: team structure, leadership, situation monitoring, mutual support, and communication (35 items).	T-TPQ Manual. http://teamstepps.ahrq.gov/Teamwork_Perception_Questionnaire.pdf Agency for Healthcare Research and Quality. TeamSTEPPS®: National Implementation. 2010. Accessed Oct 20, 2012. http://teamstepps.ahrq.gov.
Communication and Teamwork Skills (CATS) Assessment	Direct observation measures team behaviors in four categories: coordination, cooperation, situational awareness, and communication (18 items). Surgical teams. Requires validation.	Frankel A, et al. Using the Communication and Teamwork Skills (CATS) Assessment to measure health care team performance. *Jt Comm J Qual Patient Saf.* 2007 Sep;33(9):549–558.
NOn-TECHnical Skills (NOTECHS)	Measures surgical cooperation, leadership and managerial skills, situation awareness and vigilance, decision making, and communication and interaction (22 items). Surgical teams. Requires further validation.	Sevdalis N, et al. Reliability of a revised NOTECHS scale for use in surgical teams. *Am J Surg.* 2008 Aug;196(2):184–190.
Modified Collaborative Practice Scale (CPS)	Measures interdisciplinary collaboration between nurses and physicians: assertiveness and cooperativeness (13 items). Requires further validation.	Cheater FM, et al. Can a facilitated programme promote effective multidisciplinary audit in secondary care teams? An exploratory trial. *Int J Nurs Stud.* 2005 Sep;42(7):779–791.

Appendix G

WEB-BASED QUALITY AND SAFETY EDUCATION

Mary A. Dolansky

Table G-1, below, includes examples of Web-based resources for education related to quality and patient safety, which can support efforts to learn about and apply ideas for practice-based learning and improvement.

Table G-1. Web-Based Education Resources

Organization	Web Address	Description
Achieving Competence Today (ACT)	https://act.med.virginia.edu/blocks/pla/index.php	A guide for educators to help develop curricula for health care professionals
Association of American Medical Colleges (AAMC): Integrating Quality (IQ) Initiative	https://www.aamc.org/initiatives/quality/	An initiative that assists AAMC members in enhancing the culture of quality in their organization by providing resources
Healthcare Improvement Skills Center (HISC)	http://www.improvementskills.org	A website providing tools for health care professionals to improve their quality improvement skills
Institute for Healthcare Improvement Open School	http://www.ihi.org/offerings/IHIOpenSchool/Courses/Pages/default.aspx	An online school that educates health care professionals on the skills needed to become change agents in health care improvement
Joint Commission Resources	http://www.jcrinc.com	A not-for-profit affiliate of The Joint Commission (and its official publisher and educator) that offers publications, software, educational conferences and webinars, and consulting services to help health care organizations improve quality of care and patient safety
MedEdPORTAL Teaching for Quality	https://www.mededportal.org/about/initiatives/te4q/	A program sponsored by the AAMC that hosts a database of peer-reviewed teaching and faculty development materials and assessment tools that can be easily searched
Quality and Safety Education for Nurses (QSEN)	http://qsen.org	A comprehensive resource for quality and safety education for nurses

continued on next page

Organization	Web Address	Description
VanderbiltHealth.com: Quality Improvement Course	http://www.mc.vanderbilt.edu/root/ vumc.php?site=qicourse	A course that teaches health care professionals about quality improvement and how to implement quality improvement projects
Veterans Affairs National Quality Scholars Fellowship Program (VAQS)	http://vaqs.org	A fellowship that offers scholars the opportunity to be a leader while teaching methods of health care improvement
World Health Organization (WHO) Patient Safety Curriculum Guide	http://www.who.int/patientsafety/ education/curriculum/en/index.html	A guide for universities on training health care professionals about improving patient safety

Appendix H

PUBLISHING AND PRESENTING QUALITY IMPROVEMENT WORK

Standards for Quality Improvement Reporting Excellence (SQUIRE) Guidelines

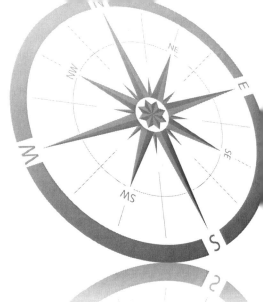

Greg S. Ogrinc

As in other fields, writing and presenting one's work help advance the field of quality improvement (QI) by disseminating proven innovations and offering the potential to reduce unnecessary or redundant work. Sharing one's QI work also can stimulate new ideas for others. But writing and presenting QI work can be challenging. Improvement work is often done by local, frontline staff members who are primarily concerned with making their care delivery better. Often these individuals have little to no experience or expertise in publishing or sharing their work. They may work for organizations that do not have incentives for publishing or presenting. Nevertheless, sharing individual QI successes (and failures) is vital to the advancement of the field.

Writing about quality improvement is particularly difficult compared to biomedical or clinical research writing. Improvement is not the same as evaluation of drugs, clinical procedures, or database analysis. Quality improvement involves complex, multicomponent interventions that may occur at many levels of an organization. The interventions are adapted and evolve in response to feedback. Change can be fragile, and results might be unstable. Uncertainty exists regarding what aspects and details of the QI work should be shared.

In 2008 the Standards for Quality Improvement Reporting Excellence (SQUIRE) guidelines were published concurrently in six biomedical journals.[1] The SQUIRE guidelines are a checklist of 19 items for reporting about quality improvement (*see* Table H-1,

pages 184–186). They are similar to other publication guidelines such as CONSORT for randomized controlled trials or STARD for diagnostic tests. The immediate purpose of SQUIRE was to increase the completeness, precision, and transparency of published reports about quality improvement. The ultimate purpose is to encourage more and better published QI reports. The target audience includes authors, editors, reviewers, funders, and improvers.

Since their publication, the SQUIRE guidelines have been adopted by dozens of journals in health care reporting. They have been used as the basis for writing the annual report for hospital QI departments, submitting abstracts to national and international conferences, and guiding prospective QI work. Full details about the guidelines, journals, and sample articles can be found on the SQUIRE website (http://www.squire-statement.org).

The guidelines provide a framework for reporting formal, planned studies designed to assess the nature and effectiveness of interventions to improve the quality and safety of care. Because the guidelines are organized in the traditional journal article format—introduction, methods, results, and discussion—they have a familiar design for authors and readers. Although each corresponding section of a published original study generally contains some information about the numbered items within that section, information about items from one section (for example, the introduction) is also often needed in other sections (for example, the discussion).

The SQUIRE guidelines attempt to balance the impact of interventions with the explanation of mechanisms for improvement. The guidelines are not intended to apply to reviews or commentaries and do not work well with rigid, mechanical use. They are not a "fill in the blank." In a manner of speaking, the SQUIRE guidelines do not clean up a messy room, but they turn on the light so that you can see what needs cleaning.

The 19 items in the SQUIRE guidelines are intended to be comprehensive for any QI work; however, they are particularly helpful for planned studies that assess interventions to improve quality and safety in specific health care settings. It is often not appropriate to include information about each and every SQUIRE item or subitem. Authors should tailor their writing to include the most important elements to convey the story of their work, but they should at least consider each item in their manuscript to ensure completeness.

Writing about QI work is challenging but important to move our field forward. The SQUIRE guidelines provide one framework for authors to organize their work and write a comprehensive manuscript that includes the most salient points. Please visit the SQUIRE website for resources. An interactive version of the guidelines is available at http://qualitysafety.bmj.com/content/17/Suppl_1/i3.long.

Reference

1. Davidoff F, et al.; SQUIRE Development Group. Publication guidelines for quality improvement in health care: Evolution of the SQUIRE project. *Qual Saf Health Care.* 2008 Oct;17 Suppl 1:i3–i9.

Table H-1. Standards for Quality Improvement Reporting Excellence

Text Section; Item Number and Name	Section Question to be Answered or Item Description
Title and Abstract	*Did you provide clear and accurate information for finding, indexing, and scanning your paper?*
1. Title	*a. Indicates that the article concerns the improvement of quality (broadly defined to include the safety, effectiveness, patient-centeredness, timeliness, efficiency, and equity of care)* *b. States the specific aim of the intervention* *c. Specifies the study method used (for example, "A qualitative study," or "A randomized cluster trial")*
2. Abstract	*Summarizes precisely all key information from various sections of the text using the abstract format of the intended publication*
Introduction	*Why did you start?*
3. Background Knowledge	*Provides a brief, nonselective summary of current knowledge of the care problem being addressed and characteristics of organizations in which it occurs*
4. Local Problem	*Describes the nature and severity of the specific local problem or system dysfunction that was addressed*
5. Intended Improvement	*a. Describes the specific aim (changes/improvements in care processes and patient outcomes) of the proposed intervention* *b. Specifies who (champions, supporters) and what (events, observations) triggered the decision to make changes, and why now (timing)*
6. Study Question	*States precisely the primary improvement-related question and any secondary questions that the study of the intervention was designed to answer*
Methods	*What did you do?*
7. Ethical Issues	*Describes ethical aspects of implementing and studying the improvement, such as privacy concerns, protection of participants' physical well-being, and potential author conflicts of interest, and how ethical concerns were addressed*

continued on next page

Table H-1. Standards for Quality Improvement Reporting Excellence, *continued*

Text Section; Item Number and Name	Section Question to be Answered or Item Description
8. Setting	*Specifies how elements of the local care environment considered most likely to influence change/improvement in the involved site or sites were identified and characterized*
9. Planning the Intervention	a. Describes the intervention and its component parts in sufficient detail that others could reproduce it b. Indicates main factors that contributed to choice of the specific intervention (for example, analysis of causes of dysfunction; matching relevant improvement experience of others with the local situation) c. Outlines initial plans for how the intervention was to be implemented: for example, what was to be done (initial steps; functions to be accomplished by those steps; how tests of change would be used to modify intervention), and by whom (intended roles, qualifications, and training of staff)
10. Planning the Study of the Intervention	a. Outlines plans for assessing how well the intervention was implemented (dose or intensity of exposure) b. Describes mechanisms by which intervention components were expected to cause changes, and plans for testing whether those mechanisms were effective c. Identifies the study design (for example, observational, quasi-experimental, experimental) chosen for measuring impact of the intervention on primary and secondary outcomes, if applicable d. Explains plans for implementing essential aspects of the chosen study design, as described in publication guidelines for specific designs, if applicable (see, for example, www.equator-network.org) e. Describes aspects of the study design that specifically concerned internal validity (integrity of the data) and external validity (generalizability)
11. Methods of Evaluation	a. Describes instruments and procedures (qualitative, quantitative, or mixed) used to assess (1) the effectiveness of implementation, (2) the contributions of intervention components and context factors to effectiveness of the intervention, and (3) primary and secondary outcomes b. Reports efforts to validate and test reliability of assessment instruments c. Explains methods used to assure data quality and adequacy (for example, blinding; repeating measurements and data extraction; training in data collection; collection of sufficient baseline measurements)
12. Analysis	*a. Provides details of qualitative and quantitative (statistical) methods used to draw inferences from the data* b. Aligns unit of analysis with level at which the intervention was implemented, if applicable c. Specifies degree of variability expected in implementation, change expected in primary outcome (effect size), and ability of study design (including size) to detect such effects d. Describes analytic methods used to demonstrate effects of time as a variable (for example, statistical process control)
<u>*Results*</u>	*What did you find?*

continued on next page

Table H-1. Standards for Quality Improvement Reporting Excellence, *continued*

Text Section; Item Number and Name	Section Question to be Answered or Item Description

13. Outcomes	a. Nature of setting and improvement intervention
	  i. Characterizes relevant elements of setting or settings (for example, geography, physical resources, organizational culture, history of change efforts), and structures and patterns of care (for example, staffing, leadership) that provided context for the intervention
	  ii. Explains the actual course of the intervention (for example, sequence of steps, events or phases; type and number of participants at key points), preferably using a time-line diagram or flowchart
	  iii. Documents degree of success in implementing intervention components
	  iv. Describes how and why the initial plan evolved, and the most important lessons learned from that evolution, particularly the effects of internal feedback from tests of change (reflexiveness)
	b. Changes in processes of care and patient outcomes associated with the intervention
	  i. Presents data on changes observed in the care delivery process
	  ii. Presents data on changes observed in measures of patient outcome (for example, morbidity, mortality, function, patient/staff satisfaction, service utilization, cost, care disparities)
	  iii. Considers benefits, harms, unexpected results, problems, failures
	  iv. Presents evidence regarding the strength of association between observed changes/ improvements and intervention components/context factors
	  v. Includes summary of missing data for intervention and outcomes

Discussion	*What do the findings mean?*
14. Summary	a. Summarizes the most important successes and difficulties in implementing intervention components, and main changes observed in care delivery and clinical outcomes b. Highlights the study's particular strengths
15. Relation to Other Evidence	*Compares and contrasts study results with relevant findings of others, drawing on broad review of the literature; use of a summary table may be helpful in building on existing evidence*
16. Limitations	a. Considers possible sources of confounding, bias, or imprecision in design, measurement, and analysis that might have affected study outcomes (internal validity) b. Explores factors that could affect generalizability (external validity), for example: representativeness of participants; effectiveness of implementation; dose-response effects; features of local care setting c. Addresses likelihood that observed gains may weaken over time and describes plans, if any, for monitoring and maintaining improvement; explicitly states if such planning was not done d. Reviews efforts made to minimize and adjust for study limitations e. Assesses the effect of study limitations on interpretation and application of results
17. Interpretation	a. Explores possible reasons for differences between observed and expected outcomes b. Draws inferences consistent with the strength of the data about causal mechanisms and size of observed changes, paying particular attention to components of the intervention and context factors that helped determine the intervention's effectiveness (or lack thereof), and types of settings in which this intervention is most likely to be effective c. Suggests steps that might be modified to improve future performance d. Reviews issues of opportunity cost and actual financial cost of the intervention
18. Conclusions	a. Considers overall practical usefulness of the intervention b. Suggests implications of this report for further studies of improvement interventions
Other Information	*Were there other factors relevant to the conduct and interpretation of the study?*
19. Funding	*Describes funding sources, if any, and role of funding organization in design, implementation, interpretation, and publication of study*

Source: Reproduced from Davidoff F, et al.; SQUIRE Development Group. Publication guidelines for quality improvement in health care: Evolution of the SQUIRE project. *Qual Saf Health Care*. 2008 Oct;17 Suppl 1:i3–i9; with permission from BMJ Publishing Group Ltd.

Index